EXECUTIVE POWERBUILDING

The Proven Strength & Muscle Building Formula for Men Over 40

by

Rex Holloway

Elite Fitness Trainer
Nutrition Coach
Bodybuilding Specialist

www.RexHollowayWriter.com

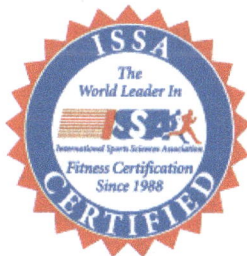

EBook: 979-8-9906572-1-2

PAPERBACK: 979-8-9906572-2-9

Front cover image by Rex Holloway

Book design by Rex Holloway

Chapter 1

PROLOGUE

About this Book

This is not a health science text, exercise technique manual, or 12-week abdominal-building program. This book is the condensed total of everything I've learned in 30-years of fitness. You're holding a combination of research, experience, and personal reflection. Most of the things you're confused about are things I've also faced and can now help you with.

Anyone of any gender or age can use this book. It presents a safe, effective, and fun approach to weightlifting suitable for anyone. That said, it is addressed to men over 40 mainly because:

1. I see a lot of guys my age coming back to the gym who want guidance; and
2. I am a man over 40, so the topics covered here concern me, too.

Men in our 40s find ourselves at a new place in life. In a lot of ways, we're doing the best we ever have. We are far enough into our careers to make a decent living. Many of us are married. Many have families. But while school, work, moving, career, family, vacations, date nights, and ball games have defined our lives for the past 20-plus years, we find ourselves facing the facts: we're not so young anymore, and things are beginning to hurt. The life expectancy of an American man is about 79 years, but we all know of guys passing away much younger. We are becoming aware of our mortality, and yet we're not quite ready to retire to our rocking chairs. Deep down, we know we have one last hoorah in us. Great news! 40 is not too late to start working on your dream body. But just as you would not enter an investment or relationship as recklessly now as you would have 20-years ago, we're going to leverage that maturity and experience and work smarter.

With this book, I propose to reduce all the confusing fitness advice out there into essential concepts that are quick and easy to deploy in your life, saving you years of mistakes, injuries, and wasted time. I already did the trial-and-error for you, so you can learn from my mistakes instead of recreating them.

About Me

I was never an elite athlete, but I was capable enough. I played the full range of sports, eventually settling on soccer as my main childhood focus. Then, during 7th grade, my school added wrestling to its athletics program, a sport that was not widely available in the Houston area in those days. I was one of the first to join the team. The trouble was, at 12- or 13-years old, I was a twig with little to no muscle development. I shot straight up in junior high, surpassing 6-feet tall but barely tipping the scale at 140-lbs. I had the heart of a strongman, but the genetics of a swimmer or cross-country runner. Every day I endured brutal, multi-hour workouts with the wrestling squad, ran for miles at soccer practice, and did barbell curls in my bedroom mirror at night, all the while picturing myself as the next Conan or Rocky. The trouble was, while I could run 2 miles in 12-minutes and do 50 push-ups straight, I was still scrawny. In wrestling, physique matters because you compete by weight class, similar to boxing. Logically, the best physique for a weight-classed athlete is one with maximum muscle (useful mass) and minimum body fat (not useful mass). Conditioning and "making weight" were drilled into my head so deeply that, even as skinny as I was, I sometimes ran 2-miles around the neighborhood in a plastic suit after practice, all the while thinking I'd be packing pecs like Arnold any day if I just worked a little harder.

Of course, it never happened. I was doing cardio and interval training for 2-or-more-hours per-day, lifting weights sporadically, and eating pizza and candy bars while avoiding nutritious food as much as possible. I had no idea what I was doing. I joined a Nautilus gym and watched the older lifters roar and spit tobacco into the trashcans, rattling the metal roof every time they dropped the barbell.

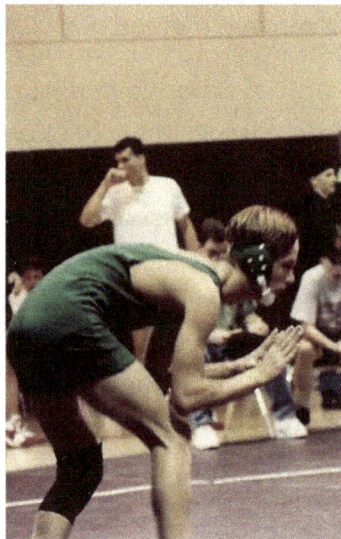

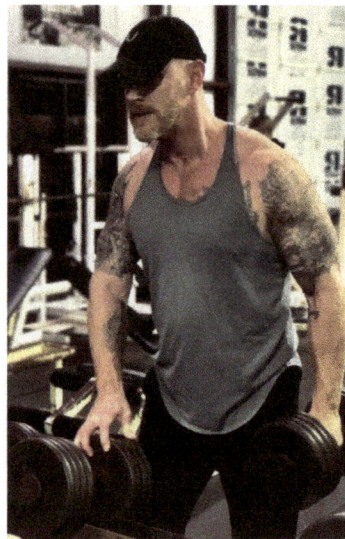

30-years and 70-lbs difference

I convinced my mom to buy me a tub of weight-gainer (which I drank whenever I remembered, not when it made sense to, so results were limited). These were pre-internet days, so fitness information was hard to come by. Somewhere in there, I learned the terms "ectomorph" and "hard gainer". I was discouraged all the time, but I didn't quit—at least not yet.

By the time I was 19, I had learned how to structure a workout, eat for gains, and progressively increase the weight I lifted to build strength. Over the next couple of years, I gained 40-pounds of muscle and finally hit my bench press goal of 315-lbs. Throughout my 20s, I read every fitness magazine I could: Muscle & Fitness, Flex, Men's Health, Men's Fitness. I followed the pro bodybuilders like Jay Cutler and Ronnie Coleman. I experimented with workouts and diets. I got deep into bodyweight exercises. At one point, I did 1,000 push-ups in 1-hour because I'd heard somewhere that Herschel Walker could do it. For a while, I thought I wanted to be a trainer, but one thing continuously bothered me: I just wasn't that big. After all the years of study and practice, I was no closer to looking like Arnold than I was a kangaroo. After years of buying supplements, working through injuries, and dreaming of rippling muscles, I was burned out.

In my late 20s, the gym took a backseat to work, and I did not return the iron pile until I was 36. Returning to regular weightlifting was a bit of a shock. First, for the first time in my life, I needed to lose weight. Second, one word: injuries. Holy cow, the injuries. I can only think of 2 gym-related injuries before I slowed down at 28. When I returned at 36, it wasn't uncommon for me to nurse 2-or-more injuries at the same time.

This proclivity to injury forced a new round of research, this time aided by the greatest resource of all time: the internet. I am a voracious reader. To rest my brain throughout the day, I take micro-breaks by reading, my favorite being fitness articles. I may read 10 fitness articles every day, and I have done so for years. The internet has done more for fitness than even Joe Weider, in my opinion. Growing up, most of the advice about gaining muscle came through some media source controlled by Joe, and his media was funded heavily by supplement, apparel, and equipment manufacturers.

There has always been that one dirty secret in bodybuilding: *everyone* is on illegal steroids. But the fitness industry wants consumers to think bodybuilders get their physiques through hard effort and proper nutrition, while supplement companies use these drug-induced physiques to market their vitamins and supplements, all of which have negligible effects on physique when compared to actual performance-enhancing drugs (PEDs). In other words, bodybuilding, like pro wrestling, is mostly an illusion. Trust me: all the creatine and whey protein on earth will never make you look like Ronnie Coleman or Jay Cutler. That was not as easy to understand back in the day when the industry controlled the fitness media, and the goal was to sell supplements. Steroids were never discussed. But it only takes a couple of years of serious lifting to realize that Arnold Schwarzenegger did not get 21-inch biceps from cheeseburgers and cheat curls. Now, the internet, with its free market for ideas, has brought forth so much accurate, factual information. Top fitness professionals and YouTubers like Jeff Cavalier and Jeff Nippard present trustworthy, scientific information about fitness—for free! The internet is an absolute goldmine of free knowledge, if you know where to look. The trouble with the internet, of course, is all the junk information. The fitness industry is all about sales, just like every other business. There is no end to the online trainers eager to tell you whatever you want to hear or parrot whatever is trending just to sell you a workout program or nutrition plan. That's where fad diets and fitness gadgets come from. They are products of an industry which needs to generate sales just like any other industry. But, for consumers, it can be hard to tell what is good fitness advice and what is not.

For that reason, I decided to put my knowledge to the test and pursue fitness training certifications so I can help people like you sort through all this fitness stuff. By completing the Fitness Trainer, Nutritionist Coach, and Bodybuilding Specialist Coach certifications, I earned ISSA's Elite Fitness Trainer title. After all these years, it was gratifying to sit down and go through the texts, verifying what I had already deduced from years of trial-and-error and self-study:

Natural bodybuilding is about long-term strategies, not tricks and cheat codes.

About My Theory

Your mind is an extension of your physical brain. Your brain is nourished and influenced by the rest of your body. The mind, brain, and body cannot function separately from each other. When one part of our body suffers, so does the rest. To truly perform at peak capacity, we must keep the entirety of our physical form in top condition. We are a holistic system, and when we neglect our body to satisfy our unreliable brain by, say, drinking too much or overeating, we end up hurting both our body and mind. It's an illogical, self-defeating loop where we crave bad things that then cause us to be unhealthy. And what's worse, it's part of who we are as a species.

Humans have been around for about 300,000-years. For 96% of that time, we were hunter-gatherers. Agriculture only evolved about 12,000-years ago—not genuinely long enough for our genes to adapt to the new diets. (That's why people in non-dairy drinking societies are lactose intolerant. They have not evolved the gene to produce lactase, which is the enzyme needed to digest cow's milk.) For 96% of human existence, scarcity was the rule, and like other animals, if ancient humans wanted food, they had to expend a lot of energy out in the wilderness to get it.

Then we developed agriculture, and the division of labor intensified, eventually leading to mass farming of food by a few to feed the many, freeing up humans to pursue ventures other than food production, such as creating better tools and technology. Less than 100-years ago, mass food production and technology collided, and we began creating processed food in factories. Food became calorically dense, nutritionally empty, spoilage-resistant, very cheap, and very addictive. Refined sugar made its way into everything. Americans eat out more now than ever, and we have fast-food restaurants on every corner. At the same time, technology allows us to live ever-more sedentary and comfortable lives. More-and-more we find ourselves sitting behind desks, hardly using our bodies. So now we, the heirs of ancient hunter-gatherers, genetically programmed to "see food, eat food," find ourselves surrounded by this vast cornucopia of delicious, cheap food while at the same time our energy needs are decreasing. No other animal has ever had such a bounty of sustenance. Even poor people are overweight in America. These days, you can order food from any restaurant for home delivery through a smartphone app. Because restaurants must compete for customers like every other business, we have food advertising. Think about that. Food is a necessity of life. We are built to be hungry. Do we really need to advertise it? Food advertising is a massively influential tease that taps into our most primal urge—the need to eat—passed down to us from generations of hungry, wandering ancestors.

In their article, "The evolution of BMI values of US adults: 1882-1986", John Kolmos and Marek Brabek wrote that more than a third of Americans are obese. They go on to identify the following causes for the increase in American obesity:

"...the "creeping" nature of the epidemic, as well as its persistence, does suggest that its roots are embedded deep in the social fabric and are nourished by a network of disparate slowly changing sources as the 20th-century US population responded to a vast array of irresistible and impersonal socio-economic and technological forces.

The most obviously persistent among these were:

- the major labor-saving technological changes of the 20th century,

- the industrial processing of food and with it the spread of fast-food eateries (To illustrate the spread of fast food culture, consider that White Castle, the first drive-in restaurant, was founded in 1921. McDonald started operation in the late 1940s, Kentucky Fried Chicken in 1952, Burger King in 1954, Pizza Hut in 1958, Taco Bell in 1962, and Subway in 1962.),

- the associated culture of consumption,

- the rise of an automobile-based way of life,

- the introduction of radio and television broadcasting,

- the increasing participation of women in the work force, and

- the IT revolution.

These elements—taken together—virtually defined American society in the 20th century."

(Kolmos, J., & Brabek, M. (2010). The evolution of BMI values of US adults: 1882-1986. Retrieved from https://voxeu.org/article/100-years-us-obesity)

In the technologically advanced Western world, we are the victims of our own success. Humans evolved to feel hunger, store energy as body fat, crave carbs, and favor rest over work. All of these attributes are logical in the context of an ancient hunter-gatherer society—but they are deadly to a modern American man who passes a dozen restaurants every time he leaves his comfortable house or office. Rapid technological advances plus lagging, outdated DNA combine to create excess body fat, diabetes, and cardiovascular disease. Since we live in an artificial ecosystem, we must consciously make decisions to maintain a healthy physical condition. We can't just eat whenever we crave food or relax any chance we get. We must consciously make plans to eat nutritious food and exercise. I have come to think of my body as an asset I must manage. Just as I make time to look over my finances and make plans for the future, just like I take my car in for preventive maintenance, just like I learn new skills to increase my value to clients, I also make time to attend to my body's physical needs. After all, I am a holistic system.

Mark Rippetoe wrote in "Starting Strength,"

> "Humans are not physically normal in the absence of hard physical effort. Exercise is not a thing we do to fix a problem—it is a thing we must do anyway, a thing without which there will always *be* problems. Exercise is the thing we must do to replicate the conditions under which our physiology was—and still is—adapted, the conditions under which we are physically normal. In other words, exercise is substitute cave-man activity, the thing we need to make our bodies, and in fact, our minds, normal in the 21st century. And merely normal, for most worthwhile humans, is not good enough." (Rippetoe, Mark (2017) *Starting Strength: Basic Barbell Training* (3rd rev. ed., pp. 1) Wichita Falls, TX: The Aasgaard Company)

Exercise is not optional. If we don't have to physically labor for our food, then we must make conscious choices to conduct healthy replacement activities instead. If not, our muscles will wither away from disuse, causing us to be weak, frail, and unhealthy far earlier in life than necessary. Only by using and straining our bodies do we even maintain good health, let alone develop an attractive, admirable physique.

But no matter how we work to maintain our bodies, age comes for everyone eventually. You can see endless examples of people keeping fit into their 80s, so we know that proper nutrition and exercise work well to reduce physical age, while a sedentary lifestyle and poor diet are linked to early physical aging. But how is fitness training at 40+ different from training at, say, 20?

First, you heal more slowly when you get older. A lot of that is due to lower testosterone levels. If you don't adjust your training to that fact, you will find yourself over-trained, burned-out, and injured. Second, a lot of grown men bring existing injuries to the gym. I have military veteran friends who bring severe pain from battle wounds to the gym. Pain is a problem a lot of men carry, and we need a strategy to deal with it. Third, as we get older, we tend to accumulate body fat more easily as our metabolisms slow down.

In my mind, there is a certain yin and yang balance in nature that must be respected. Times of intense activity must be followed by times of rest and recovery. This up-and-down motion, or undulation, is key to long-lasting success in the gym, especially for the older trainee. Staying lean given reduced capacity to heal requires a different approach than just training harder-and-harder to burn more-and-more calories. Training after 40 takes a more nuanced approach, something we will cover thoroughly in the pages ahead.

About My System

Once we realize that our bodies operate on a "use it or lose it" basis and that nobody ever spontaneously got in shape sitting on their butt, then we know we must take action. What action, though? There are many ways to be "in shape." A powerlifter and a marathon runner, a swimmer and a sprinter, all can be said to be "in shape", just in different ways, as their personal preferences and needs guide them. More to the point, their *training* is very different.

This book is about getting "in shape" in a particular way called "powerbuilding."

- **Powerbuilding** is a hybrid weightlifting system that combines powerlifting and bodybuilding techniques to enhance both strength and physique synergistically.

Is powerbuilding better than other ways of training? That's the wrong question. It's the wrong way to train if you want to improve your time in a triathlon. But it's the right way to train if you want to get strong and muscular over the age of 40. Your goals guide your choice of training. Just like when I was a kid on the wrestling squad, whose goal was to gain muscle yet spent most of my time doing cardio, a mismatch between goals and training methods will yield disappointing results. If your goal is to get bigger and stronger, then powerbuilding is the best training technique available.

Let's dig deeper into this concept of "powerbuilding." First, let's break the word apart. Clearly, it's a portmanteau of "powerlifting" and "bodybuilding," so let's look at those two separately.

- **Powerlifting** is a weightlifting method that seeks to increase skeletal muscle limit strength.

- **Bodybuilding** is a weightlifting method that seeks to increase muscle size and reduce body fat for aesthetic purposes.

Combined, we deduce that powerbuilding is then a modality by which we seek to improve both strength and appearance in coordination.

Now here's an important point I want you to take away: I draw a line between the *activities* of powerlifting and bodybuilding and the *competitive sports* of powerlifting and bodybuilding. One can be a bodybuilder and never step on stage. One can be a powerlifter and have no intent to compete. Competition is not the defining attribute of the sports, but rather the goals and the activities that support those goals are what define powerlifting and bodybuilding. A powerlifter is someone who seeks to increase their physical strength by executing the "Big Lifts"—bench press, deadlift, squat, and overhead press. Bodybuilders seek to improve their physical appearance by building muscle and losing body fat. Anyone can do these activities whether or not they compete.

I think this is what most guys want to achieve when they join a gym—to improve both strength and appearance. But what they often don't realize is those two don't always build together at the same time. Increasing strength and muscle mass both require adequate food intake (a caloric surplus) while losing body fat to reveal the muscles underneath requires eating fewer calories than needed (a caloric deficit). Trying to gain strength and muscle while also losing fat at the same time is equivalent to pushing and pulling simultaneously, leaving the trainee stuck in neutral or, worse yet, injured. In order to build strength *and* muscle *and* lose body fat requires a smart, patient, and holistic approach, and this is especially true for men over 40.

When we were in our teens and our metabolisms and testosterone were the highest they'll ever be, when we played sports or were out-and-about as much as possible, our bodies were much different than they are now. Gaining muscle and strength after 40 is absolutely doable, but there are a few things we have to be conscious of, like slower recovery and a slower metabolism. Once we take everything into account, we can design a complete system that will get us to our goals under real-world conditions. Another laughable "21-Day Plan to Get Super Ripped!" or smoothie recipe book is not going to cut it. We need a complete system covering mental, physical, and nutritional concerns specific to the man over 40, and that's what this book provides.

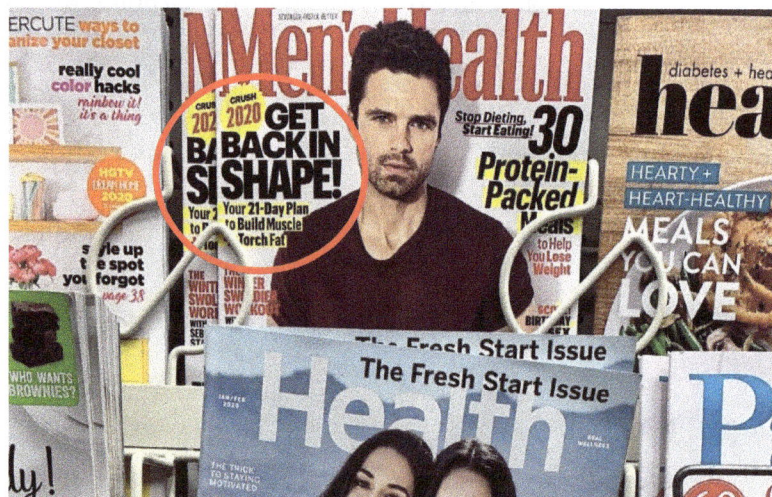

What's lacking in the world of fitness advice is not more workout programs. Those are a dime a dozen. What trainees are missing is the Big Picture. Trust me: you don't want to learn to deadlift from a book. It would be better for you to watch 10 YouTube videos on how to deadlift or hire a trainer to coach you in person than for me to clog the bookshelves with yet another book on some tedious exercise detail. Natural bodybuilding is about long-term strategies, not one or two technique tricks.

At the same time, you don't need to know the Krebs cycle or how to label the organelles of a cell to understand how to influence changes in your body. With this book, I will take all the confusing details of fitness and simplify them to just the right level for a man of your abilities.

Chapter 2

MENTAL

Mental Essentials

When people hire trainers, they often want someone to motivate them. That is, they want *external motivation*. I'm quick to say that I don't even believe in external motivation. Instead of trying to motivate someone to do something they should want to do on their own, I would rather teach them to motivate themselves. Make no mistake; our attitudes about exercise affect our success. If you dread working out or hate your nutrition plan, then you will not succeed. Fitness should not be a drag. In fact, it should be a joy. If you don't enjoy your program, you won't stick with it long enough to achieve your goals.

In my view, motivation stems from knowledge. That is, when we know what we ought to do, then we are confident in taking action. It's when we are uncertain if the planned course of action will be effective that we hesitate. Faith comes from knowledge, and faith generates motivation. But motivation is fleeting and unreliable. If we had to rely on motivation to get up every morning for work, we would likely be out of a job. Instead of motivation, we rely on discipline to get us up and going every day, day-after-day, because we believe that the effort is (a) necessary for survival, and (b) will bring a better lifestyle later. The discipline to get up and go to work every day is what carries us through to the big promotions and eventually, hopefully, wealth and comfortable retirement. That is a great analogy for what it takes to build a bigger, stronger physique.

Let's break this down. We need 3 mental aspects to succeed in fitness. They are:

- **Knowledge**

- **Motivation**

- **Discipline.**

Let's look at these independently, and then see how they interact. First, we'll set some simple definitions for each:

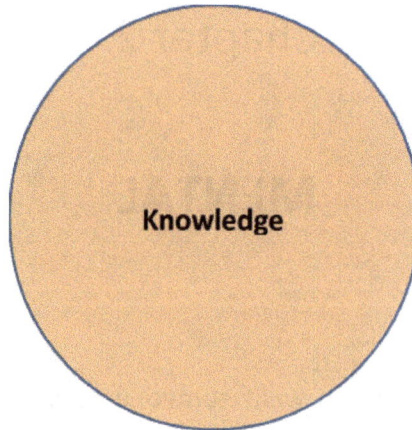

Knowledge

Knowledge

Our definition:

> **Possession and comprehension of the minimum information necessary to complete a task correctly.**

Knowledge is essential to the success of any endeavor. You don't have to be an expert, but you could be way off in your approach and therefore getting predictably poor results. This is true of anything, but especially when you're talking about coaxing a complex biological machine (your body) to improve. It's not going to be as simple as "drink green tea and do interval training." No matter how badly we want the cheat code to fitness, it just doesn't exist. People have been programmed by decades of fitness industry marketing that getting in top shape is a matter of collecting all the right cheat codes (drink lemon juice, put butter in your coffee, meditate more) or unlocking the latest exciting health secret (inevitably another fad diet, supplement, or gadget). They think it's about tricks and techniques, but it's not. Honest trainers and nutritionists have been saying it all along, but their voices get drowned out by millions of dollars in advertising money. We have to put those bad ideas to rest. If your fitness endeavors are to be successful, you absolutely must have the right knowledge.

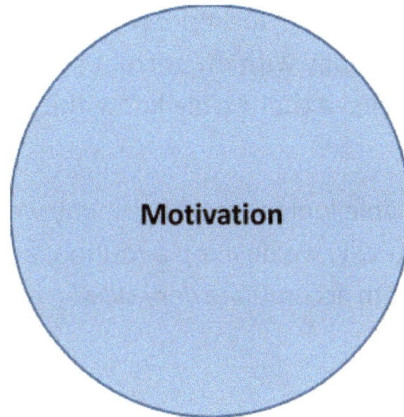

Motivation

Motivation

Our definition:

> **A feeling that can arise when we intensely contemplate an action for which the expected benefits outweigh the expected costs.**

Motivation is the most over-used, unproductive word in fitness. How many books, articles, and memes have been created about motivation? There are numerous competing theories about motivation, each of which has value in different fields and to different people. But to self-motivated men—to *bosses*—motivation is not generally a problem. After all, you've been getting up and taking care of business your whole life, right? We don't need to look into theories about internal and external motivation. We just need to analyze what you already do and apply it to fitness.

How is it that you get up every day and go to work? Do you lay in bed and debate about getting up? Do you think, "I don't feel like going today," and just call it in? I don't think so; otherwise, you'd be out of a job, right? At this point in life, you just get up and go because it's routine. But how did it become routine? Think back to younger days. Maybe you knew what you wanted to do when you were a kid. Maybe it didn't hit you until later. Once you knew what you wanted to do with your career, next, you learned what steps to take in order to achieve that goal, which may have included enrolling in school, taking an internship or apprenticeship, or starting at the bottom and working your way up. It took real effort to get where you are, and I'm sure at times it was a real struggle. But you kept going. Why? Because you believed that if you followed the right steps, you would eventually land the job you wanted, which will, in turn, lead to the lifestyle you want. Every day of school, training, or apprenticeship, grinding away at entry-level and hoping to improve your lot in life, took faith because those are not the days when you're motivated by the actual cash compensation you receive. A young man's days are spent paying his dues, working hard for little because of a promised pay-out later in life. That feeling that kept you going—that motivation—came from a combination of deeply wanting to succeed and faith that you were taking the right steps. That is, your motivation ultimately arises from the possession of (a) a core, emotional need to improve your current state, and (b) the correct knowledge to fill that need. If I am happy with my current state or uncertain what to do about it, I will be hesitant to act. But if I believe that I truly know the way to improve my life, I will feel confident to act.

But motivation is a fleeting, unreliable fuel source. That's why we can't rely on motivation to keep us going to work every day. Eventually, we develop a routine, and we just get up and go because it's what we do. Muscle and strength accumulate very slowly, much more slowly than motivation alone can attain.

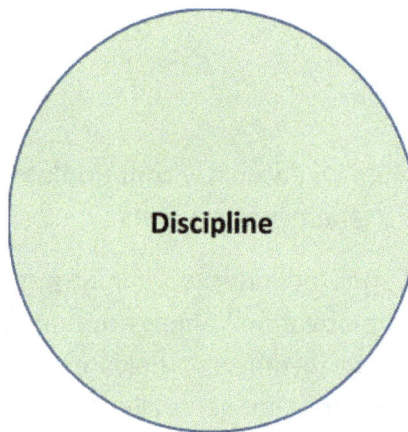

Discipline

Our Definition:

The ability to maintain a routine for a long time.

Discipline trumps motivation in the long run. Imagine you're at home. Maybe you just got off work, maybe your alarm just went off at 5:00 am—either way, it's gym time, and you know it. If you begin having that debate, "Do I really want to go?" you are setting yourself up for failure. I tell trainees, "Don't think about it. Just do it!" Set your workout schedule and stick to it with the exact same dedication you have for your professional schedule. After all, is your financial health more important than your actual health? By repeatedly executing an action, you develop a routine that becomes completely natural. Discipline alone has the endurance needed to build an impressive physique.

The KMD Dynamic

In summary, knowledge leads to motivation, and over time, we develop a routine that sustains us for the long haul. But what happens if we find ourselves quitting the program? Why do so many people quit working out after just a few weeks or months? The theory described above that relates knowledge, motivation, and discipline can be used to diagnose why we might lose our determination to get in shape.

Let's look at how the separate concepts of knowledge, motivation, and discipline interact with each other and see what happens when a piece is missing.

The KMD Dynamic

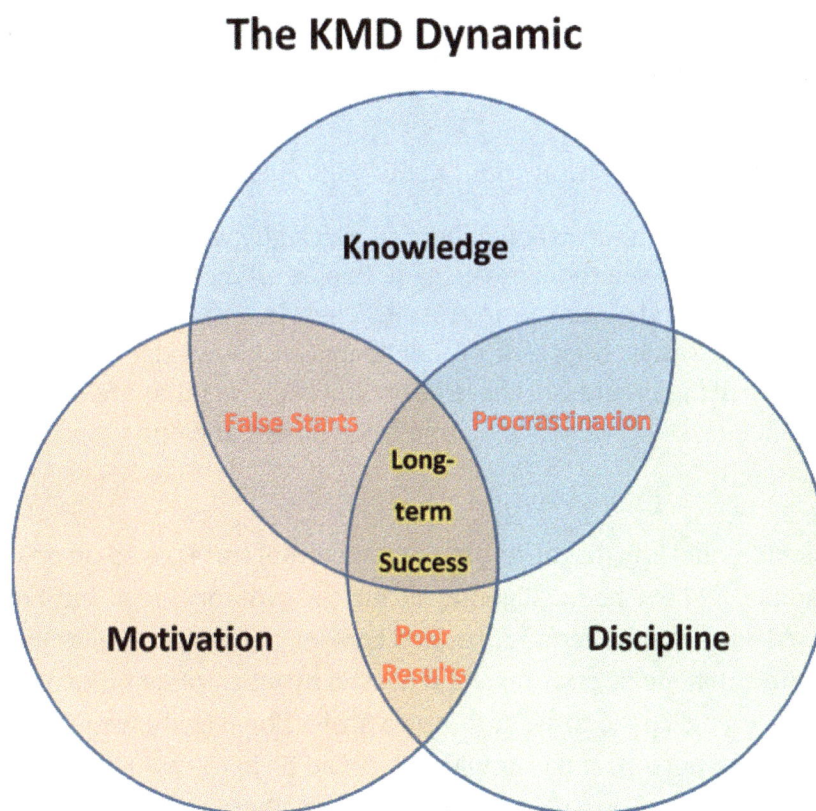

In the Venn diagram above, we notice that where all 3 elements—knowledge, motivation, and discipline—intersect, we achieve long-term success.

But what happens when we're missing one of those key elements? In those cases, we see various types of failures.

For instance, we see that:

- Knowledge *plus* Motivation *but without* Discipline leads to **false starts**

This is because motivation is a short-term emotional response. It's temporary excitement, a flash in the pan. This is what leads people to join a gym, buy all new workout clothes, and then quit going after a few weeks. That's a false start. Nothing lasting is accomplished in such short periods of excitement.

We also see that:

- Knowledge *plus* Discipline *but without* Motivation leads to **procrastination**

This is the case of someone who knows what he *should* do, someone who is generally a disciplined person, but for some reason, he does not feel compelled to act *right now*. I've been this guy before. I knew that I should be exercising, and I'm generally a disciplined person, but I just wasn't feeling it at the time. Burned out. Uncaring. Distracted by life. Having knowledge and being a disciplined person is not enough. We usually can't reason our way into the gym. We need motivation. To take that first step and say, "Today's the day!" we usually need that spark of emotion.

- Discipline *plus* Motivation *but without* Knowledge leads to **poor results**

This describes the case of the well-meaning, hard-working guy who just doesn't know what he's supposed to be doing. We all see them at the gym. People who come in and do their not-quite-right routine day-after-day and never see any results. There's no lack of determination or effort—which is admirable—but rather a lack of proper technical knowledge. We must differentiate "staying busy" with "making progress." There are many exercises that are inefficient, and if you don't have the Big Picture, it's easy to slip on one key element and end up with poor results.

Diagnostic Use

The real power in this model is in diagnosing your own mental state based on objective, observed behavior. For example, if I have been diligently hitting the gym for a year, but I'm still not seeing results, then I would diagnose that as poor results. Looking at the KMD Dynamic Venn diagram, I see that diligent effort that yields poor results is caused by incomplete or incorrect knowledge. I am doing something wrong. I need to study or hire a professional to show me the right way. What if I know I'm a disciplined person, and I know that I should be in the gym, but I just never go, day-after-day? For some reason, I keep procrastinating about going to the gym. Why? Because I'm missing that emotional spark necessary to get me going. Maybe I'm just not that down on how I look or feel. Maybe it just doesn't seem *that* fun to work out compared to other activities in my life. If I'm going to fix this procrastination problem and get my butt into the gym, I'm going to have to figure out why I'm running so lukewarm on the subject.

You get the idea. If you're in the gym getting results, that means you're right in that center sweet spot of the KMD Dynamic, with all elements playing their part. But if you find yourself failing in the gym, or failing even to go, then step back and take an assessment of your mental state, determine which element is missing—knowledge, motivation, or discipline—and work on it. Once you bring that lagging aspect up, you'll be excited to hit the gym, and the results will follow.

Bridging the Gap

The KMD Dynamic would be of limited real-world value if it was a static model; in other words, if it didn't take into account, change through time. Over the years, I've had numerous workout partners and trainees, and what I've learned is there are two kinds: (1) the ones who show up and stick with it, and (2) the ones who quit in less than 90 days. Rough guess, I would say the population splits about 50/50 on the two types. What happens is their motivation runs out before discipline can kick in. For a behavior like going to the gym every Monday, Wednesday, and Friday, to become routine requires sufficient repetition. If you only do something a few times, it is unlikely to imprint as a new behavior pattern.

I call the time between the fire of initial motivation and the establishment of an actual routine "The Gap." Whenever somebody I'm training starts off with big goals and determination but drops off after a few weeks or months, I say they "fell into the gap." And that's what it is—a no-man's-land between the excitement of a new gym member's first days and the days farther down the road when actual gains become visible. People get discouraged in between those points, plain and simple. Working out does eventually become fun, but it is hard in the beginning, especially to someone who's never really lifted. Add to that the unrealistic goals that new trainees often bring to the gym, influenced by years of dishonest fitness advertising, and they get bummed when they don't "Get ripped in just 30 days!" as they'd hoped. It's deflating and discouraging. They also have other things in their life competing for their free time, such as family, hobbies, and side businesses.

The Gap

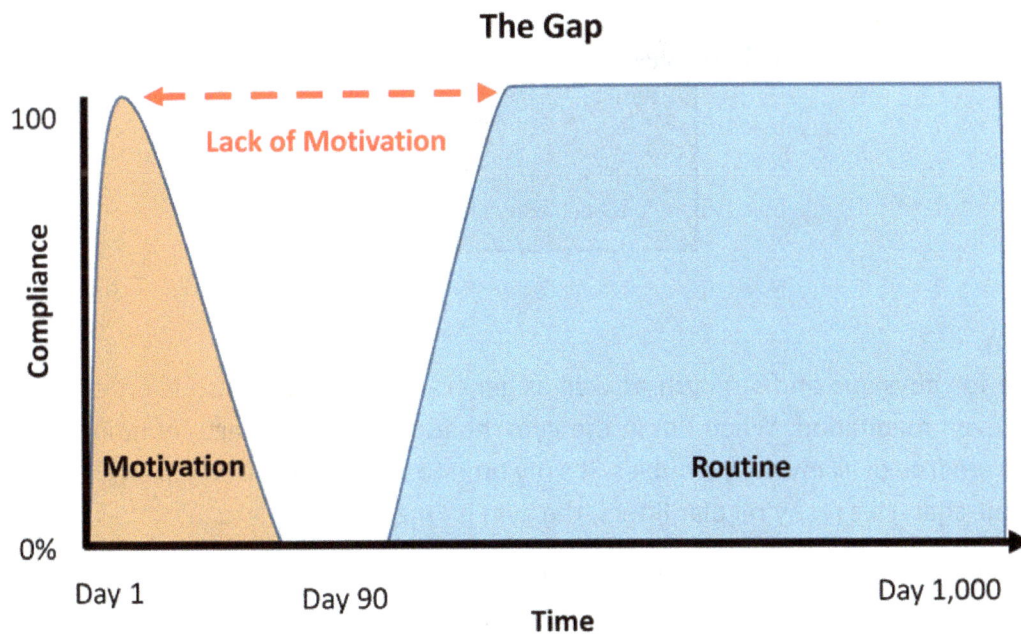

Many a good man has fallen into The Gap. What we need is a solution for powering-through times of low motivation, especially before a stable routine has been established. The trick, if you will, is to look to short-term results for verification that your efforts are working and draw renewed motivation from those little victories along the way. Let's face it: building a muscular physique takes 2-10 years of effort, depending on the trainee. The pay-out is far enough in the future that it can get discouraging along the way. Once we've plotted an overall course, it is best then to set short-term goals (3-6 months out) and focus on those instead of obsessing over something that can't be rushed.

Powerbuilding is a patient, persistent man's game—but it's mostly an illusion of patience. People who train seriously have an overarching, long-term goal, sure. But instead of obsessing over that distant goal, they find enjoyment now by hitting short-term goals. With most new trainees or people coming back to the gym after a long period off, the first gains are in strength. I like to test a new trainee's ability to perform a few basic exercises. How much can you deadlift? Now work to add 90-lbs to that number. How many push-ups can you do? Set a goal to double that. Can you do a pull-up? No? Why not say, "I'm going to work until I can do 10 pull-ups straight," and work on that? These are goals that can be reached in weeks or months instead of years. Fill your life with victories, even small ones, and you will always find a renewed drive. Bridge "The Gap" by stringing together short-term victories, and one day you will make it across to your ultimate goal.

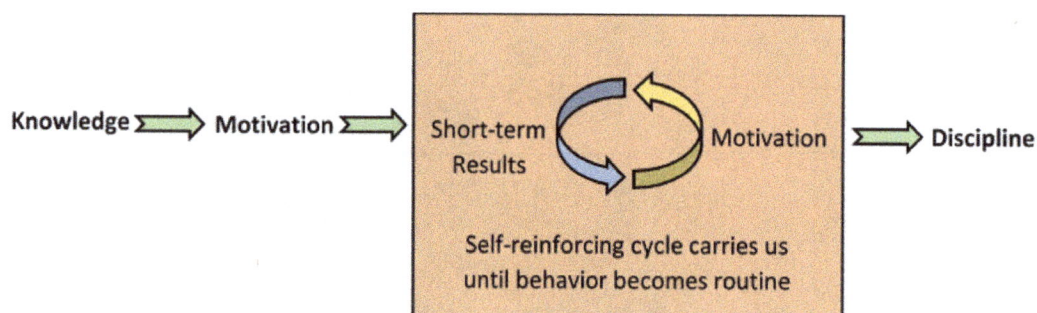

Knowledge ⇒ Motivation ⇒ | Short-term Results ⟲ Motivation ⇒ Discipline

Self-reinforcing cycle carries us until behavior becomes routine

Gym Zen

I exercise for physique and strength as well as general health. But I also exercise as a form of therapy, even meditation. When I'm in the gym, headphones on, heart pounding and muscles burning, I am free of all my daily troubles. It's my time to let it all go. I don't like workout partners or gym chit-chat. Like many regular lifters, the gym is "me" time.

When we exercise, our bodies release feel-good hormones called endorphins. These pleasure hormones serve as a reward for doing something positive for yourself. When they're really flowing, you get a detached, almost floating feeling. I call all of this Gym Zen, and in time, it becomes as important to a lifter's well-being as the exercise itself. Don't feel bad about going to the gym and zoning out, forgetting your troubles, and ignoring everything and everyone except yourself and the next set.

Essential Takeaways

- Knowledge, motivation, and discipline are all required to build a strong, muscular physique.

- If you find yourself procrastinating, quitting, or getting poor results, use the KMD Dynamic to diagnose what's missing and fix it.

- Motivation is unreliable. Only discipline will carry you for the long-haul.

- Use short-term (3-6 months) goals to power through times of low-motivation, especially before discipline kicks-in.

Chapter 3

FUNDAMENTALS OF POWERBUILDING

Powerbuilding Essentials

In powerbuilding, we have a three-part goal:

1. Build strength
2. Build muscle
3. Lose body fat

When we talk about a ripped physique, we're talking about body composition. Body composition is essentially the ratio of muscle-to-body fat we carry. When we talk about a **recomposition** or **recomp**, we're talking about reducing body fat and increasing muscle mass. If we want to appear muscular, we need to build and shape the muscles, but also reduce body fat so the muscular definition can be seen. The classic analogy to describe the effect body fat has on muscle definition is, "Place a tennis ball under a thin, cotton bed sheet and note how pronounced the ball appears. Next, place a down comforter on top of the ball. Can you still clearly see its shape?" While powerlifting is strictly about pounds lifted, bodybuilding is about aesthetics. It's about building muscle, yes, but it is equally about developing a balanced, lean physique with visible muscle definition. Excess body fat is undesirable to the bodybuilder. So how do we go about attaining the goal of a lean, strong, and muscular body?

First, you have to understand one of the most important rules of exercise:

You get what you train for.

The International Sports Sciences Association (ISSA) identifies seven "Granddaddy Laws" of training, all of which must be adhered to, but one, in particular, bears special attention. It is called the SAID Principle, which stands for Specific Adaptation to Imposed Demands. The ISSA has this to say about SAID:

"If your training objectives include becoming more explosive, then you have to train explosively. If you desire greater limit strength (primarily from an increase in the cross section of myofibrils), you must use heavier weights than if you were training, for example, local muscular endurance (capillarization and mitochondrial adaptation). If your objectives include deriving cardiovascular benefits, then you must tax the heart muscle as well as the oxygen-using abilities of the working muscles.

In fact, the SAID principle is so uncompromising in its highly researched tenet of training "specifically" that problems frequently arise if one possesses more than one training objective at a time. <u>The specific training required for one will frequently detract from the expected gains in the other. For example, training for aerobic strength endurance (aerobic power) will severely limit the level of strength one can attain.</u>"

(Hatfield, Frederick C., Ph.D. (2018) *Fitness: The Complete Guide* (9th ed., pp. 418) Carpinteria, CA: ISSA)

The SAID principle says that if you run a lot, you'll get better at running—and that's really it. If you do a lot of push-ups, the muscles involved in pushing (mainly chest, shoulders, and triceps) will simply get better at performing that repetitive movement pattern, but it won't make you a better runner. Your body adapts specifically to the strain placed upon it to better deal with that strain in the future. It strives to be more efficient. But building bulky muscle is not helpful in becoming a better long-distance runner, so your body has no need to create a bunch of new muscle in response to daily jogging. Instead, the muscles of your heart will strengthen, and your body will sprout new capillaries to distribute oxygen-rich red blood cells to your muscles since more oxygen is needed to run farther, not more skeletal muscle strength. You get what you train for.

In fact, there isn't just one type of muscle or one type of muscle fiber (the contractile structures that makeup muscles). There are generally 2 different types of skeletal muscle fibers:

- **Type I** are slow-twitch fibers mainly used in long endurance activities, like jogging. They are efficient at using oxygen for fuel and clearing out waste. They have a high resistance to fatigue, but their force output is low.
- **Type II** are fast-twitch fibers mainly used in strength and power activities, like weightlifting. They have a fairly low resistance to fatigue but a high force output.

Exercises that mainly utilize Type I muscle fibers will not make your muscles larger because Type I fibers don't really get bigger, or **hypertrophy**. They just get more efficient. Type II fibers are the ones used for weightlifting. They are the ones that can be coaxed into growing larger. So, if you want bigger muscles, running 5-miles before breakfast isn't going to help.

Instead, to grow bigger muscles, you must strain your Type II fibers. One way to accomplish this is to push your weightlifting sessions harder-and-harder over time, a key concept of powerbuilding called **progressive overload**.

- **Progressive overload**: The gradual increase of stress on the body through exercise.

- **Supercompensation**: A muscle's adaptation to progressive overload.

For powerbuilders, progressive overload can be accomplished in more than one way. They are:

- **Increase Intensity**: Increase the weight lifted over time.

- **Increase Volume**: Increase sets and/or reps over time.

- **Increase Density**: Decrease rest breaks between sets over time.

- **Increase Tension**: Increase the time it takes to complete each rep over time.

An advanced powerbuilder knows how to mix these techniques to get the best results. While ultimately the goal is to lift more weight—that is, to "increase intensity," as the pros say—as you'll see below, there are times when it is actually better to use one of the other techniques, such as reducing weight but increasing sets and reps, known as "increasing volume." There is a line when increasing volume, though. If you drop the weight so low, you can do almost endless reps of, say, dumbbell shoulder presses, then you are probably not straining the Type II muscle fibers in your shoulders. Instead, you are taxing your Type I fibers and, therefore, only building endurance. It's like jogging for your shoulders. Your muscles don't have to get bigger to jog farther. You get what you train for.

I learned this lesson the hard way from years of doing thousands of push-ups, pull-ups, and bodyweight squats, but not getting any bigger. There was nothing genetically wrong with me; my fitness knowledge was just wrong. I had learned from athletics coaches to do calisthenics, so that's what I did. But that style of training was never going to build muscles bigger than absolutely necessary to lift my body weight. To get bigger, ultimately, I needed to lift heavier weights than just my bodyweight. That doesn't mean there is no place for lighter-weight, high-rep work. It is a valid technique for overloading your body. You just have to know when, how, and why to use the different overload techniques, and that's something we're going to cover.

Hypertrophy

Let's just get this out of the way: I know you are here for sleeve-busting guns, slug-stopping pecs, and a back you could land an F-14 on. Big muscles are the first things we think of when we hear "bodybuilder." This is the realm of muscular hypertrophy.

- **Hypertrophy**: An increase in muscle size.

There are two types of muscular hypertrophy:

- **Myofibrillar hypertrophy**: an increase in the size and structure of muscle fibers. This type of hypertrophy is mainly accomplished through high weight, low rep training. This type of training is also associated with denser, thicker muscles.

- **Sarcoplasmic hypertrophy**: an accumulation of noncontractile muscle elements such as water, glycogen, and mitochondria in the muscle cells. This type of hypertrophy is increased through high-rep, moderate-weight training.

You know that pumped feeling your muscles get when you lift, especially when you perform a lot of reps? That "gym pump," as it's known, is short-term sarcoplasmic hypertrophy caused by an increase of blood in the muscles. While myofibrillar hypertrophy is an increase in the actual muscle tissue (picture a rubber balloon), sarcoplasmic hypertrophy is more like the water in the balloon. What's important and interesting is that *both* types of hypertrophy are necessary to achieve a muscular, bodybuilder-type physique, so we must train for both. Since we see the two types of hypertrophy are trained differently, the SAID principle dictates that we must train for them separately.

Strength

Two of the biggest names in bodybuilding, Arnold Schwarzenegger and Ronnie Coleman, started as powerlifters before winning multiple Mr. Olympia titles each as bodybuilders. So, it can't be impossible to train for size and strength at the same time, right? And progressive overload means that as the months and years go by, a trainee must get stronger in order to get bigger, right?

Yes, that's right. But strength is not simply a factor of muscle size. Looking at powerlifting records can be a real eye-opener. American powerlifter Taylor Atwood stands just 5'6" and weighs 163-lbs. As of this writing (2020), he holds the International Powerlifting Federation record in his weight class for squat—a whopping 622.6-lbs. How can someone so small lift nearly 4 times his bodyweight? It turns out, strength is more a result of the density of neurons in the muscles rather than simply the cross-sectional size of the muscle. For this reason, we call increases in strength **neurological adaptations**. This is how smaller powerlifters can out-lift huge bodybuilders. It's also how people pull off heroic feats of strength, like heaving a car or boulder off a trapped person. Your **central nervous system (CNS)** has immense electricity-generating power, and it's those electrical pulses sent out across your neurological system that cause your muscles to contract with force. More muscle fibers twitching at once causes stronger contractions, and the body's ability to fire off those fibers is limited by the number of neurons in the muscle. The muscle fibers—or more correctly, the motor units—are like electrical machines. They can do great work, but only if they're plugged in and switched on. And the more juice you can provide them, the more work they can perform.

Now, this is where you might be a little confused. Earlier in this book, I said that increasing intensity, or weight on the bar, is a way to get bigger. Now I'm saying that lifting heavier-and-heavier weights only coaxes our nervous system to adapt by laying out new neurons. What gives? Now you see the relationship between size and strength is not so straightforward as "increase one and the other will follow." It takes many inputs to build bigger muscles, not just putting additional strain on your muscles.

In a later chapter, we will talk about strategies and tactics for getting stronger, and in the grand scheme of things, as you get stronger, you will also get bigger. But that is because we will treat strength as a complementary but separate adaptation from muscle size. In other words, we build them both, just not at the same time. We will divide our year into phases, or "cycles," where we work on just one of the desired goals—strength, hypertrophy, or fat loss—at a time, and then bring them all together at the end in one strong, ripped package.

Body Composition

Most people cannot gain muscle *and* gain strength *and* lose body fat at the same time, especially not the steroid-free, natural bodybuilder-of-a-certain-age. Now, I know there are plenty of fantastic trainers and scientists who will argue that you absolutely *can* gain muscle and lose fat at the same time. Of course, that sounds great because that's what we *want* to hear. I'm not saying it's biologically impossible. I'm saying most likely it will not work for you, that it will be a waste of time to try, and that there is a better way.

Let me put it like this:

You can't increase body mass *and* decrease body mass at the same time.

Gaining muscle means gaining weight. Gaining body mass requires a **caloric surplus**, meaning you must eat more than your body needs in total; that is, enough to cover all of its normal, daily functions *plus* building new tissue. In a purely biological sense, food provides us with two things: (1) nutrients and (2) energy. The structures of our bodies—our bones, eyes, nerves, skin, muscle, and so on—are all built from the nutrients we eat. To build up more body tissue requires an influx of more building material—that is, more nutrients from food. It's all quite mechanical, really.

Losing body mass, such as belly fat, on the other hand, requires a **caloric deficit**, meaning you must eat less food than your body needs to function. When your body is starved for fuel because you're burning more calories than you're eating, your body must turn to its own internal energy stores—body fat—to supplement its energy needs. That's the entire science behind losing body fat, in a nutshell. Again, it's intuitive, really.

Now consider this:

You cannot be in a caloric surplus *and* a caloric deficit at the same time.

That's just logical. Then how do we build both a lean *and* muscular physique? Is it all hopeless without steroids? No, it's not hopeless. We just have to be smart about it. Once we understand the basic rules, we can devise a strategy that actually works in the real world.

The tried-and-true strategy for building a ripped physique naturally involves cycling between periods of muscle gain, called **bulk phases**, and periods of fat loss, called **cut phases**.

- **Bulk Phase**: A period of high caloric intake paired with intense weightlifting with the goal of building muscle while minimizing body fat accumulation

- **Cut Phase**: A period of low caloric intake and lighter weightlifting and cardio with the goal of reducing body fat while preserving muscle

By cycling between bulk and cut phases, we can effectively work towards each goal set without conflict.

The ability to shed body fat while simultaneously building muscle is generally limited to men who are (a) young (high testosterone), (b) new to training (so-called "newbie gains"), (c) are very overweight when they start training (they may have enough body fat stored to fuel their own gains), or (d) are on PEDs. I struggled with this dilemma in my youth before I learned better. I wanted to increase muscle mass while also carving a six-pack at the same time. Even at that younger age, it was a pointless struggle. You are effectively pushing and pulling at the same time and therefore getting nowhere. In fact, trying to lift heavy while in a caloric deficit leads to injuries, as your system is underpowered to handle the weight. Every injury I've ever sustained in the gym has occurred while I was cutting calories. It is far safer to cycle between bulking and cutting phases so that you never try to lift the heavy weight while undernourished. When I'm cutting, I reduce weight on the bar and increase reps and sets to keep the workload up. That has proven to be a successful, safe strategy.

It's important to realize that cardio and weightlifting both compete for available resources. I admit, I really don't care ever to jog again. A lot of that comes from years of stagnant gains due to over-training, a result of doing cardio and bodybuilding workouts within the same week in an attempt to get big, cut, strong, and well-conditioned all at once. Mostly, what I got was a disappointment. You see, it comes down to the way new muscle is built.

When we exercise, we create **micro-traumas** within our bodies—little bits of muscle and tendon damage that must be healed, and preferably upgraded and improved. That's why we work out, after all. Exercise causes microtrauma, and when you rest, your body goes to work repairing them. These repairs are physical, even mechanical. They require energy, raw materials, and capable workers, just like building any physical structure. In this analogy, the energy and raw materials you need are provided by the food you eat, and the capable workers are your hormones that guide and regulate the repair activities. If you're not eating enough to support both the repair activities *and* your normal bodily functions, then some work within your body is going to be incomplete. And if you keep doing this—taxing your body and then not giving it enough fuel and materials to repair itself—all the partially completed work within your body will accumulate, and your body will start scavenging itself for raw materials to repair the damage. When your body is borrowing from Peter to pay Paul by taking protein from one muscle to repair another, guess what your net gain is? A wash, nothing, nada.

Not every bit of food you eat is available for building new muscle. Most of the food you consume—in fact, about 70% of it as measured in calories—will go towards fueling basic bodily functions, such as keeping your heart beating, your brain sizzling, and your bowels mushing. These are calories you would burn even if you were in a coma because keeping a complex human body functioning is a massive undertaking. In order to keep all those processes humming while also building additional tissue (such as muscle mass) requires additional resources. The more you break your body down in exercise, the more you need to eat to build it back up.

But this is a dangerous oversimplification. We're missing a crucial element, and one I want to really drive home to you as a 40+ lifter. It's not as simple as, "The more you lift, the more you can eat, and therefore the faster you'll get big muscles." Not so fast.

Think of it like this:

1. You lift weights, thereby creating microtrauma in your muscles, which must be healed using fuel and nutrients from food.
2. At the same time, your brain, heart, lungs, etc. must still function, and they also require fuel and nutrients.
3. You eat a meal after your workout.
4. Now that your body has fresh new supplies to divvy out to the bodily systems, how does the body decide where and how to allocate those resources?

I imagine a tiny economy inside the human body where different systems must compete for whatever resources are available. If there is not enough food coming in to fulfill all bodily needs, then some systems must suffer. You simply cannot run at optimal capacity if you are starved for oxygen, water, or food. But what if it was a big meal; that is, what if there was a surplus of energy and nutrients? Only some of the nutrients can be used to repair muscle and tendon damage at any given time. Any excess over what the body can use gets excreted or stored as body fat—an undesirable result. If the secret to muscle growth is causing microtrauma and then eating in excess so your body can repair itself and grow, then simply working out more and stuffing your face would seem to be the strategy for maximizing gains. But in reality, your body's capacity to repair and grow is limited by several factors—primarily your genetics, age, and testosterone levels. Your body has its own ideas about how much muscle tissue it can repair at any given time and how much excess energy it wants to store as body fat. Some people are more genetically inclined to lean muscle growth (**mesomorphs**), some are more inclined to body fat accumulation (**endomorphs**), and some struggle to gain a pound of anything (**ectomorphs**).

We don't fully understand what it means to say someone is "genetically gifted" as a bodybuilder because we don't know all the biological secrets of muscle building. We know that some people simply have more Type II muscle fibers than others, which means they have a greater capacity for hypertrophy. We also know that certain hormones, especially testosterone, greatly increase muscle size and strength, even without exercise. This is the power of **anabolic/androgenic steroids (AAS)**, such as exogenous testosterone. If you inject three-or-more times your natural amount of testosterone and then exercise, you will lose body fat and gain muscle at a much faster pace than you would without those injections. There is no question about that. You will also get bigger, more muscular, and leaner than you could without them. That's how pro bodybuilders can blow up to 300-or-more pounds of ripped muscle, far bigger than their natural size would ever allow, weights or no weights. They achieve this by supplementing their normal hormones with massive doses of additional hormones and drugs whose jobs are to signal the creation of more muscle tissue. But without these additional hormones, simply lifting more and eating bigger will not speed up the muscle growth process. You will just wear yourself out and gain body fat. You need the additional hormones to put all those extra calories to work.

Unique to you at your current age, and given your current testosterone level, there is a peak amount of damage you can do to your body, beyond which it will not be able to heal in time for your next workout. This natural limit is called **Maximum Recoverable Volume (MRV)**. Exceeding your body's ability to repair itself is called over-training, and **over-training syndrome (OTS)** is a real thing. When you're over-trained, your body is slowly breaking itself down because you're under-feeding and/or under-resting it. Learning things like your MRV and your maximum and minimum calorie targets are part of learning the uniqueness of your body and how to improve it.

Assume you came to me and said you wanted a bigger, stronger chest. I write you a killer chest program and tell you it'll take 5-years of consistent lifting to build the pecs you dream of. Now let's pretend 5-years is too long for you. You want the chest of your dreams in time for your trip to the Caribbean in just a few weeks. What could you do to speed the process up? Well, assume the program has you working your pecs for 2-hours each week. Quick math tells you that's about 104 hours of chest work per-year (2-hours per-week times 52-weeks per-year), so after 5-years, you will have performed 104 x 5 = 520-hours of chest work. Does it then follow that if 520-hours of work is the key to unlocking a bigger chest that if you just cram those hours into a shorter period, the results will come faster? Take it to the extreme: Couldn't you just do a single, 520-hour, 22-day chest workout and have massive pecs at the end? Don't you wish! We know from life experience that there is a limit to the amount of work we can do in a single day, both physically and neurologically. We're not diesel engines. Over time, as your body grows stronger and more efficient, your work capacity will increase. But we will always have a physical work limit, and then we must rest. We will always have to split that 520-hours of chest work into discrete cycles of work and rest to allow our bodies time to heal and grow. Be patient.

Measuring Body Fat

Over the years, I have learned many ways to measure or estimate body fat. I'm only going to tell you my favorites. There are others, but they are inferior to the ones below for one reason or another. I especially advise you not to trust bioelectrical impedance analysis (BIA) devices.

- **DEXA Scan:** This is by far my favorite and what I would call the current gold standard. Clinics that offer DEXA scans are popping up everywhere, and they are pretty affordable. I usually get scanned twice a year, and it costs about $80 each time. It's a quick (30-minutes tops), easy, non-invasive process. You lay on a bed and a scanner head zig-zags back-and-forth over you for a few minutes. The scanner can differentiate between bone, muscle, and fat tissue and calculate how much of each you have. If you're going to pay for professional body fat measurement, go with DEXA.

- **Navy Tape Measure Test:** I like this one because you can do it at home very easily. You just need a bathroom scale and a tailor's tape measure, one of those cloth tapes used for sewing. They cost about $2.00 on Amazon. Once you have those tools, go online and search for the "Navy Tape Measure Test". There are numerous online calculators you can enter your measurements into, and they will estimate your body fat.

- **Visual Estimation:** One of the easiest and most accurate ways to assess your body composition is to compare your current appearance with an array of photos depicting men at different body fat levels. Go online and search for "body fat images men" and then look at the results. There are many collages to choose from. You can get a surprisingly accurate estimate of your body fat by just looking at those.

The Truth About Abs

We can't talk about body composition without talking about that most overrated of all masculine fitness goals: washboard abs. As your body fat percentage gets lower, the layer of subcutaneous fat covering your entire body gets thinner, revealing more of the muscle definition underneath. In bodybuilding, we draw a distinction between visible muscle separations and muscle striations.

- **Muscle separation**: When the boundaries between different muscles and heads of the same muscle are visible under the skin.

- **Muscle striation**: When the boundaries between bundles of muscle fibers are visible under the skin.

Most men carry the majority of their excess body fat in their belly, lower back, hips, and thighs. The fat layer naturally gets thinner as it radiates out to the extremities, all but disappearing at the wrists and ankles. But everyone carries their body fat differently and loses it differently. We've all seen men with some definition in their shoulders and arms, despite also having a big gut. This is due to how fat is naturally distributed in their body.

That said, visible abdominal muscle separation occurs for most men at around 10% body fat. Muscle striations like you see on a competitive bodybuilding stage appear at around 4% body fat. You will learn that cutting down to 10% body fat is a major feat in itself and that 4% is best left to the pros. Sub-10% body fat, especially for men over 40, is an unnaturally low percentage. It takes long, hard, consistent effort to get that lean, and once you do, it takes the same effort to stay there. At such low body fat levels, you will probably feel weak and hungry. You will also look skinny in your clothes, and people will probably comment on your weight loss (and not necessarily in a good way). You can end up looking unhealthy, even skeletal. And for what? How often do people see you with your shirt off? Who will even know or care that you have visible abs? In my experience, women don't even care that much. You could do all that suffering for abs just to discover they didn't improve your life the way you thought.

I have found a sweet spot right around 12-15% body fat where my waist is tiny, my abs show a little, but I look full and healthy instead of thin and depleted. Find the body fat percentage that works for you—with or without abs.

Growth, Maintenance, Cut

Clearly, there are factors at play beyond just "eat big, lift big, get big." As it turns out, we are merely absentee owners, or maybe silent partners, in the daily operations of our bodies. While we might make executive decisions about what or how much to eat, we each have skilled workers inside of us—hormones—that manage our bodies on our behalf. Ultimately, our hormones have the final say what happens with the nutrients we consume. You could hit the gym hard, really wear yourself out, then go home and shovel food into your face, and, yes, you will probably gain muscle over time like that. But you will most likely gain excess body fat, too. Unless you're a veteran bodybuilder, someone who has spent years tracking calories and jockeying their weight up and down intentionally, then you will not likely know how to calculate your caloric needs accurately enough to hit that very precise, very slim caloric surplus that would allow you to gain muscle but not body fat. Also, when you're over 40, your testosterone and metabolism have both decreased, so your body has a tendency to divert energy to storage—that is, to body fat—much more than when you were young.

So, the danger in overeating, thinking it will lead to quicker gains, is you will quickly gain body fat, which in turn obscures the muscle underneath. This is an undesirable result in the long-term because the ultimate goal is a physique that shows muscle definition. But excess body fat accumulation is undesirable in the short-term, too, because you will eventually want to lose it, and doing so requires a caloric deficit. Being in a caloric deficit means a shortage of nutrients, which means your body starts scavenging from itself for fuel. What can happen during a fat-loss diet is the dieter will lose not just body fat, but lean muscle, too. Yes, your body will break down its own muscle tissue and use the protein to make energy, if needed. This can be very disheartening. I have lost a year of gains in just a few months of dieting too hard. The common prescription for maintaining muscle mass during a cut phase is to continue lifting weights during the cut. In fact, the common advice is to make sure you lift the same weight as you lifted *before* the cut, back when you were eating sufficient calories. For example, if you were bench pressing 225-lbs when you were bulking and eating 3,000 kCal per-day, then keep benching 225-lbs even when you cut calories down to 1,800 kCal per day to lose fat. The thinking is that your body only built what muscle it has because you forced it to adapt to the additional strain placed on it in the gym, and if that strain should stop, then your body will not maintain the unneeded and biologically expensive muscle tissue any longer than necessary. Use it or lose it, in other words. The trouble is, we build muscle by damaging the muscle fibers and letting it heal back. As I said above, if there are not enough nutrients available to repair the damage, then the damage will not be completely repaired, and there certainly won't be excess nutrients to build more tissue. Again, the problem is compounded in our case by age because more-and-more our bodies want to divert calories away from muscle growth and towards body fat storage. So, that one hypothetical branch of the nutrient stream that dependably fed muscle growth throughout our youth is getting thinner-and-thinner as we get older. Advice like, "Maintain intensity during a cut," is great for much younger guys and trainees on PEDs. But for the drug-free, 40+ powerbuilder, you will find your bench press drop noticeably while cutting calories. If you try to fight through it and lift heavy weights during a caloric deficit, your muscles, tendons, and joints will pay the price.

All of this sounds confusing, this dividing of nutrients and energy and repairing muscle versus storing body fat, so I'm going to teach you a simple way to understand this. I call it the **Growth, Maintenance, Cut (GMC) Matrix**. It is a simple, intuitive way of understanding all the ideas discussed above without having to get into biophysics.

Let's look at it now:

GMC MATRIX

Body Mass*	Calories	Strength
Increase	Surplus	Increase
No change	Maintenance	No change
Decrease	Deficit	Decrease

* Includes both muscle and body fat

Each colored block in the GMC Matrix forms a band. There is only one rule to the GMC Matrix:

Items within each band may only be combined with other items in the same band.

Let's see an example:

Body Mass	Calories	Strength
Increase	Surplus	Increase
No change	Maintenance	No change
Decrease	Deficit	Decrease

This combination follows the rule, so it is allowed. This is because decreased caloric intake supports decreased body mass and strength, as we discussed above.

Now, let's look at another example:

Body Mass	Calories	Strength
Increase	Surplus	Increase
No change	Maintenance	No change
Decrease	Deficit	Decrease

This combination is not allowed because decreased calories do not support increased body mass and strength. In other words, you can't eat in a caloric surplus to gain strength and lose body fat at the same time. You can't eat more and expect to lose weight or eat less and expect to get stronger. To get effective results, whether the goal is to increase muscle size or lose body fat, you must operate within the correct band. When you make your fitness plans, know what your goal is and, therefore, what band you need to be functioning in. Generally, you will always be either bulking or cutting.

Now to summarize:

GROWTH BAND
- Lift big, eat big, get big
- Gaining strength and adding muscle require a caloric surplus
- With a caloric surplus comes body fat

MAINTENANCE BAND
- If bodyweight and/or strength do not change for 2-3 weeks, a plateau has been reached
- Must change diet or workout to continue making progress

CUTTING BAND
- Losing body fat requires a caloric deficit
- A caloric deficit will also impact strength and recovery
- Reduce weight and volume to avoid injury and overtraining syndrome

Another consequence of the GMC Matrix is if there is a number of calories that will make us gain weight, and a quantity that will cause us to lose weight, then logically there must be some number of calories that is exactly equal to our daily needs. We call this **maintenance calories** or "eating at maintenance." Eating at maintenance is not necessarily a good thing, as it means we are neither gaining muscle nor losing fat, and as bodybuilders, we should always be doing one or the other. Saying your "eating at maintenance" is more of a diagnosis—a deduction we make about our behavior when we don't record any changes in our body mass. In other words, if my stated goal is to gain muscle, and if after following my plan and weighing myself for 2-3 weeks, I don't see any weight gain or loss, then I must be eating at maintenance. Since eating at maintenance does not put me in the growth band, then I know that I must increase calories if I want to increase my weight.

Set Point Weight
This problem of getting stuck at a certain weight bears further discussion. In training, there is a concept of a **set point weight**.

- **Set point weight**: the weight your body prefers to be at.

If you lose weight, it's fairly easy to gain the weight back to your set point weight. At the same time, the only way to hold excess mass above that weight is to eat excessively. This weight where your body sits most comfortably, in my experience, will also be associated with a certain body fat percentage, and both of these tend to increase little-by-little as we get older. That is to say, as we get older, our bodies tend to get heavier and fatter, and it gets progressively harder to nudge our bodies from that weight. I call this resistance to change in body mass **Metabolic Inertia**.

Bodyweight isn't stable in the short-run (day-to-day fluctuations of 2-5-lbs are normal) or in the long-run (as we get older and heavier). It's always changing. But as bodybuilders, we want to harness that change, to control and guide it. If I want to decrease my body fat, I need to consume fewer calories than I need to function throughout the day. That way, my body will look to stored energy—body fat—to supply its remaining fuel needs. But *how much* less should I eat? Enter the world of **calorie math**.

Basic calorie math is built on the assumption that 1-lb of body fat contains 3,500 kCal of energy. Therefore, to burn 1-lb of body fat per week, I would need to consume 3,500 kCal less in that week than I need. Since there are 7-days in a week, then -3,500 kCal ÷ 7-days = -500 kCal. In other words, if I eat 500 kCal per-day less than my maintenance calories, then I should lose 1-lb per week. That would work fine if it were not for the body's tendency to return to its set point weight, or more accurately, set point weight range (5-pounds or so either way). While a 500 kCal per-day deficit should be enough to create 1-lb of weight loss per-week, our bodies can be more stubborn than that, and we often find that a deeper deficit of 700-900 kCal per-day is necessary to really move the needle.

It's nothing to panic about if your weight does not immediately budge while trying to cut. Cut an additional 200 kCal per day for a week and see what that does. If still no movement, cut 200 kCal more. I have personally run greater than 1,000 kCal per-day deficits for weeks at a time, and in my experience, it caused me to lose too much muscle. I think the sweet spot for fat loss without suffering too much incidental muscle loss is a caloric deficit of between 500-900 kCal per-day, but it does depend on your body.

Adaptive Thermogenesis

Another problem is that of **adaptive thermogenesis**. I will be fair and state that the idea is unproven in humans, but it's widely believed to be true in fitness circles. Adaptive thermogenesis is the idea that the longer you eat in a caloric deficit and the leaner you get, the slower your metabolism gets. While a 500 kCal per-day deficit may have worked when you first started cutting, now it's not sufficient anymore because your metabolism has slowed to accommodate the reduced caloric environment. Science is still out on this, but I've seen what certainly appears to be slowed metabolisms in trainees who had eaten restricted calorie diets for 6 months or more. What happens is, after dieting for so long, cutting calories more doesn't cause further weight loss. The standard prescription for improving metabolism and reignite fat loss is actually to increase calories to a maintenance level and increase physical activity for a period (usually 4 weeks or so). Sometimes, trainees will lose weight even after increasing calories, which is likely due mostly to increased physical activity but also possibly to reviving their sluggish metabolisms.

Other possible explanations might exist for a **weight loss plateau**, which is defined as 3 weeks without further weight loss. The most common, I assume, is actually behavioral: forgetting to reduce calories further after losing weight. Your caloric needs are proportionate to your body weight. Once you lose weight and get smaller, your body requires fewer calories to maintain. As you get smaller, to keep a 500-or-greater kCal per-day deficit, you need to adjust your total daily calories down to match your new weight.

A conclusion of the GMC Matrix is that for any given body weight, there must be a maintenance calorie level. As you lose body weight, if you don't further reduce calories to keep pace, eventually your falling weight will intersect that maintenance calorie level you are eating, and your weight loss will stop. As you get smaller, that 500 kCal deficit gets smaller until it vanishes, and you're at a new, lower maintenance level that matches your new lower body weight—and you're stuck. In order to maintain a consistent caloric deficit, a good rule of thumb is to re-weigh yourself and recalculate your caloric needs every 2-weeks. But you should never eat less than 1200 kCal per-day, and if you find yourself barely eating but not losing more weight, consider taking a diet break and letting your system readjust.

As you get leaner-and-leaner, it gets harder-and-harder to lose more weight. "Losing the last 10-lbs", meaning the last few pounds before abs really pop, is a dreaded phrase in fitness circles. If you begin your diet at a high body fat percentage of, say, 30% or more, the fat will come off quickly and easily at first. But as you get closer to 10% body fat, you will probably see your weight loss stall. This is represented in the Metabolic Inertia graphic below. Getting leaner is like trying to push the blue ball to the left. The further you push it, the more vertically it moves up the incline, making it harder-and-harder to push. The ball really just wants to roll back to the middle—the set point range. Another conclusion from the graphic is that eating more-and-more will not lead to a linear increase in muscle gains.

Metabolic Inertia

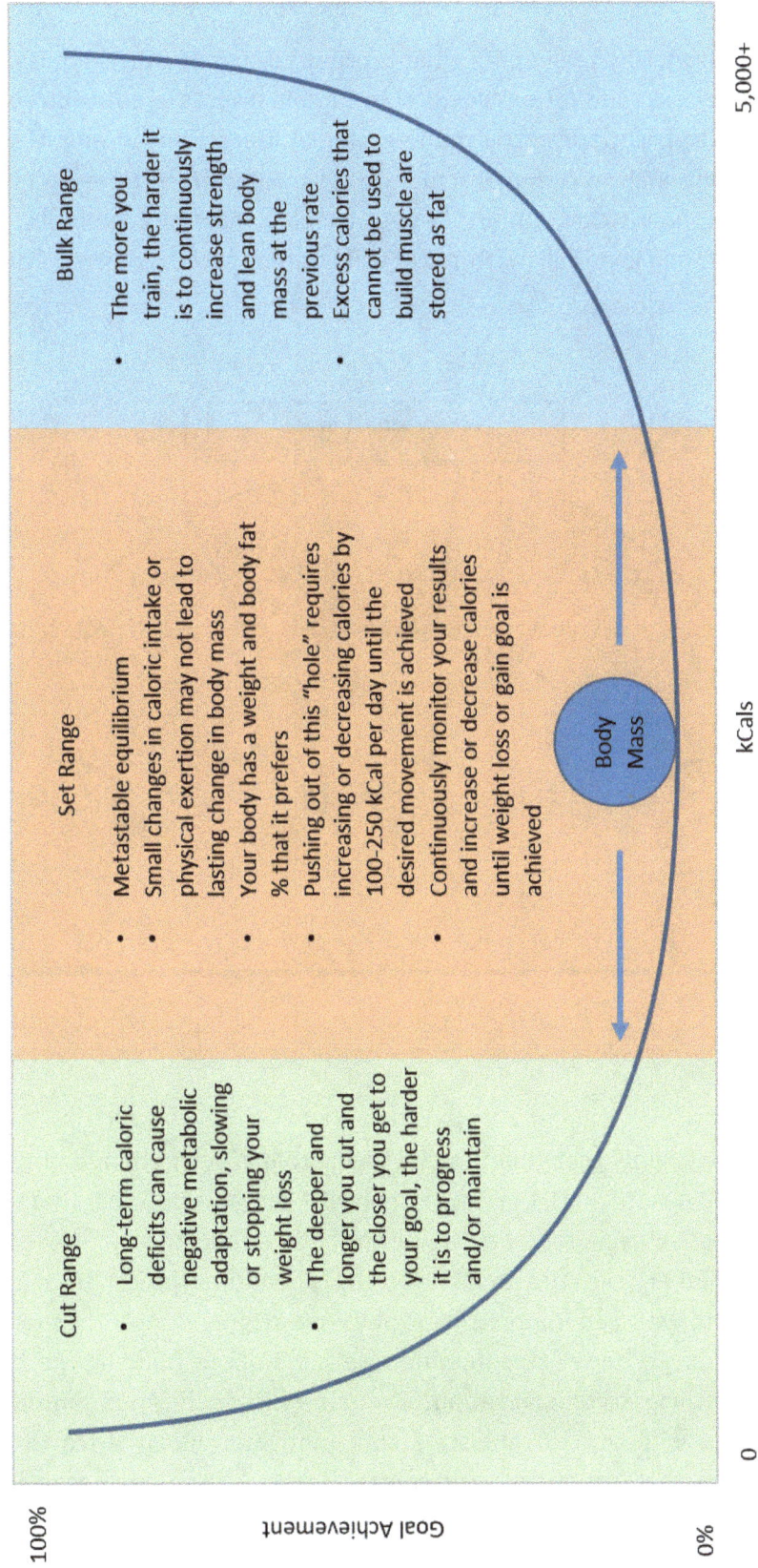

Cut Range

- Long-term caloric deficits can cause negative metabolic adaptation, slowing or stopping your weight loss
- The deeper and longer you cut and the closer you get to your goal, the harder it is to progress and/or maintain

Set Range

- Metastable equilibrium
- Small changes in caloric intake or physical exertion may not lead to lasting change in body mass
- Your body has a weight and body fat % that it prefers
- Pushing out of this "hole" requires increasing or decreasing calories by 100-250 kCal per day until the desired movement is achieved
- Continuously monitor your results and increase or decrease calories until weight loss or gain goal is achieved

Bulk Range

- The more you train, the harder it is to continuously increase strength and lean body mass at the previous rate
- Excess calories that cannot be used to build muscle are stored as fat

Body Mass

Goal Achievement

100%

0%

kCals

0

5,000+

Growth Arch

But again, I don't want to oversimplify what is required to gain muscle mass. It takes more than just modulating calories and lifting weights. In fact, it takes the contributions of many inputs. Lean muscle growth is supported by many essential inputs, and if any of those elements are missing, like a stone arch, the entire structure falls. How much time you have invested, how consistent you are, how smart you are in your training, your age, genetics, the quality of your diet, and your hormone levels all matter. We will address each of these in this book.

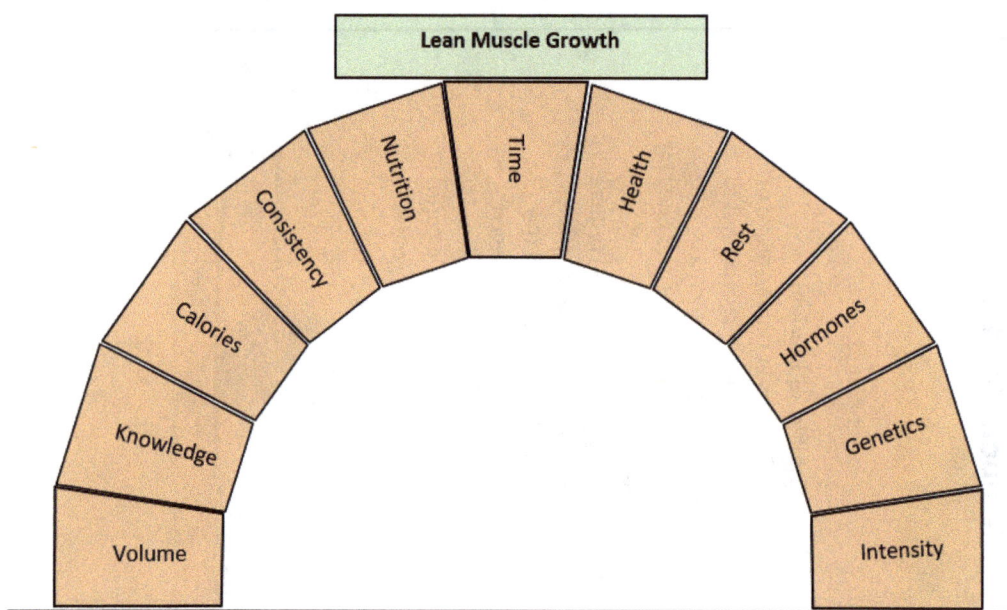

Genetic Limits

From experience, we know that genetics plays a big role in strength and physique development. If you've ever stood next to an NFL lineman or an NBA player, you know that not all men are born equal. Some men get muscle for free, like hitting the genetic lottery. There is no use in cursing your genetics. Whether you tend to gain fat easily (endomorph) or have a hard time gaining muscle (ectomorph), you can improve your physique tremendously through diet and exercise. It's not about building a body like someone else's. It's about building the best version of you. Everyone has something to complain about. Everyone wishes they had something better. It's that very dissatisfaction with our current state that motivates us to strive for more. Don't bash yourself over things that are out of your control. Instead, use your desire for improvement as motivation.

That said, Dr. Casey Butt researched the body measurements of 300 champion natural (steroid-free) bodybuilders from 1947 to 2010. From his research, he was able to deduce a formula that can estimate the maximum, drug-free lean body mass a man can hope to accumulate in his life. It turns out, the most significant predictor of maximum muscle gain is your bone structure, specifically your height, ankle circumference, and wrist circumference. Dr. Butts also created an online calculator you can use to estimate your own maximum body dimensions here:

http://www.weightrainer.net/bodypred.html

As others have pointed out, Dr. Butt's research included champion bodybuilders, representing the very elite of genetic potential, and likely included some bodybuilders who actually did use steroids. Therefore, assume the results of his calculator are probably skewed high. It makes sense to reduce those estimates by 5% or so.

I encourage you to read more about Dr. Butts work here:

http://www.weightrainer.net/potential.html

Essential Takeaways

- You get what you train for.

- Alternate between cut phases and bulk phases because you can't gain mass and lose mass at the same time.

- Expect to lose some strength and a few pounds of muscle on a cut. To minimize this effect, keep protein consumption high and don't exceed a roughly 900 kCal per day deficit.

- If you cut too deep for too long, you might find it increasingly difficult to lose weight. If so, increase your calories back to maintenance and increase physical activity a little, especially non-exercise activity, for a few weeks and then try to cut calories again, but gradually.

- If your weight won't budge at a 500 kCal per-day deficit or surplus, increase or decrease daily intake by 200 kCal per-day and check your weight again a week or two later. If it still isn't moving, add or subtract additional calories.

- There are many inputs necessary to create a strong, muscular physique. If your results are lacking over time, sit down and take an objective assessment of what you're doing and not doing. Try to identify the weakness in your Growth Arch and address it as much as possible. A lot of times, the thing holding you back is the one thing you are most resistant to change. In my experience, diet is the hardest thing for men to change.

Chapter 4

UNDULATING PERIODIZATION

Periodization Essentials

I have always been self-employed, which has made me a project-oriented person. Every project starts with a plan. Building a muscular physique is a project, in my view. A project begins at the present state and ends once the goal state is achieved. I think that's how most people approach strength training: with an image of how they want to look. What we need to do is take that future goal and work our way backward from there to where we are now, determining every step we'll need to take along the way.

Before continuing, I want to stress that the same effort it takes to build a physique is required to keep it. Please don't think that once you put in a few years of consistent work and get some nice results that you can go back to beer and hot wings and somehow keep your new body. Of course, it doesn't work that way. In that sense, building a strong body is not a project with a completion point. It's never complete because you have to maintain it. But don't let that bother you now. By the time you build your dream body, you will have established new, healthy habits, and you will never be the same again. You will eat healthily and exercise regularly because once you know, there is no unknowing. Once you're hooked, you're hooked.

So, picture your ideal body and call that the goal. Now, let's start with that goal and work backward to create a plan to get there. This is the same thing we do when planning a road trip. You must first decide where you want to go before deciding which route to take. In planning our route, we need to take into consideration the fundamental concepts we discussed earlier. How do we put all those ideas to use? For example, the GMC Matrix teaches us that we shouldn't try to lose fat and gain muscle at the same time, so over the course of the project, we need to work towards those goals separately. We know that we must take time to heal and rest to avoid injury, over-training, and allow for growth. You should be getting a distinct sense of up and down cycles by now.

Periodization means varying your workouts over time to get complete results. We talked earlier about cycling between bulking and cutting, and now we're going to really expand that idea to encompass the entire project.

- **Undulating Periodization**: an exercise strategy that alternates between cycles of high and low intensity over time.

Undulating periodization allows for:

- The parallel development of adaptations (strength, hypertrophy, and fat loss)

- Adequate deloading to avoid injury.

- Exercise variety for greater enjoyment.

Periodization in fitness involves breaking your training into discrete periods called macrocycles, mesocycles, and microcycles. Every cycle has a stated goal. Think of them as the short-term projects we talked about using as motivation in the chapter on mental state.

Macrocycles
- Duration: Entire exercise period; typically, 1 year.
- Goal: To increase strength and muscle mass and decrease body fat.

The macrocycle is the larger, overarching plan. It's the 40,000-foot view. A macrocycle could be any amount of time, but we're going to set ours to 1-year. Throughout a year-long macrocycle, you might go through several bulk/cut cycles.

Most guys come to me carrying excess body fat. There are numerous reasons to tackle that problem first, so we start with a cut phase. Over time, what happens is this:

1. Trainee cuts calories and loses body weight for a few months.

2. Trainee eventually hits a weight-loss plateau, gets bored with dieting, or decides he wants to switch to building muscle.

3. Trainee switches to a bulk cycle, eating more and lifting harder for a few months.

4. Trainee eventually gains too much body fat.

5. Trainee switches back to a cut for a while to get his body fat in check again.

And on-and-on, back-and-forth for as long as the trainee continues to train. At the end of every bulk/cut cycle, the trainee is left with more-and-more lean muscle mass. All the zig-zagging of calories, exercise, and body weight causes the whole system to trend higher over time due to lean muscle accumulation.

The diagram below depicts a basic, hypothetical 3-year period that has been divided into 6-month bulk/cut phases to demonstrate the idea.

3 CONSECUTIVE 12-MONTH MACROCYCLES

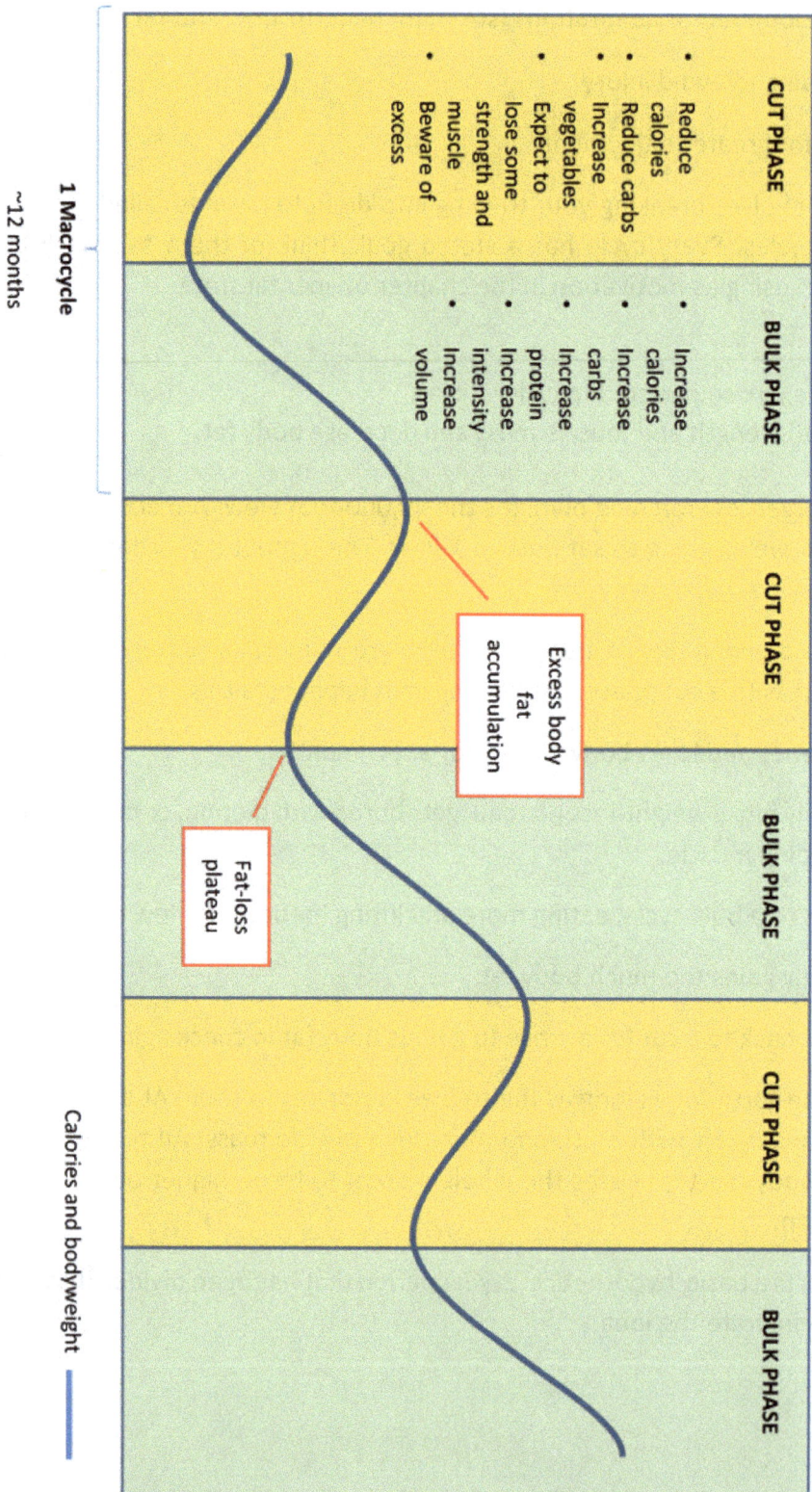

CUT PHASE
- Reduce calories
- Reduce carbs
- Increase vegetables
- Expect to lose some strength and muscle
- Beware of excess

BULK PHASE
- Increase calories
- Increase carbs
- Increase protein
- Increase intensity
- Increase volume

CUT PHASE

BULK PHASE

CUT PHASE

BULK PHASE

Excess body fat accumulation

Fat-loss plateau

1 Macrocycle

~12 months

Calories and bodyweight ——

Cycling between bulking and cutting is a common, tried-and-true method for natural bodybuilding. Even though every consumer-grade fitness plan out there would have you believe they can help you gain muscle and lose fat at the same time—and in just a few short weeks!—meanwhile, the pros are cycling between bulking and cutting. It's about as much a pro tip as I can give you, for all the reasons we talked about before.

The chart below shows the actual results achieved by one 40-year-old man during an almost 1-year bulk/cut macrocycle. He started at 211.6-lbs with about 16% body fat, which is not bad at all, to begin with, making additional weight loss more difficult. But he still managed to diet down to 194-lbs in just 5 months. At that point, his weight loss stagnated, so he switched to a bulk phase for the next 6 months. When this macrocycle ended, he had net gained 5-lbs of muscle and lost another percentage point of body fat. The route was not a straight line, but we made it to the destination of a bigger, stronger, leaner body.

RESULTS OF 11-MONTH MACROCYCLE

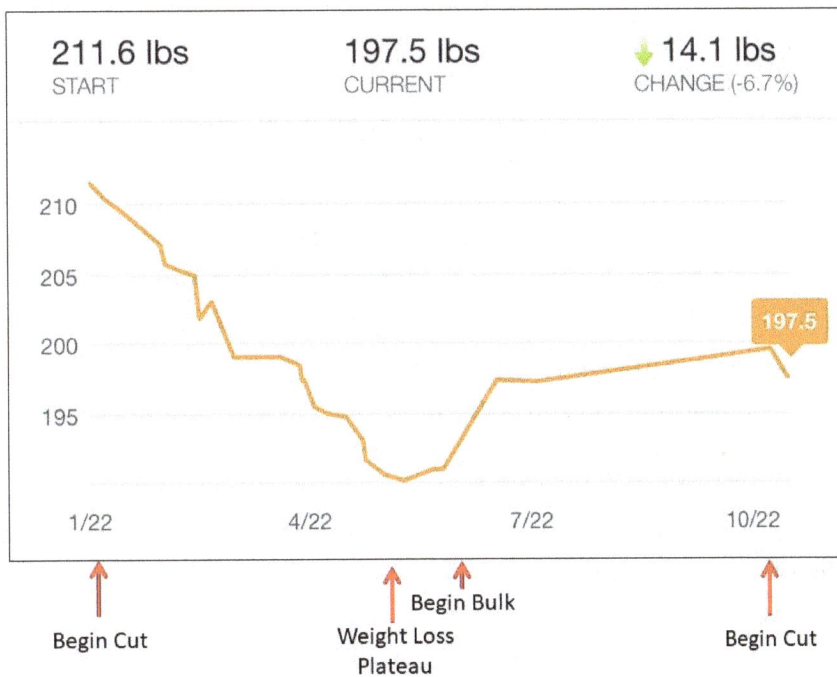

	DexaScan Measurement Date		Change	
	5/24/2018	11/27/2018	Change (lbs)	Change (%)
Total Mass (lbs)	193.7	197.6	3.90	2.01%
Lean Mass (lbs)	155.3	160.4	5.10	3.28%
Fat (lbs)	30.7	29.5	-1.20	-3.91%
Body Fat %	15.90%	14.90%		

Mesocycles

- Duration: 3-4 months each, typically
- Goal: Work on a specific adaptation, such as cutting fat or gaining lean mass

Macrocycles are broken into shorter periods called mesocycles, each of which lasts a few months. Mesocycles also have stated goals. A "6-month bulk phase to gain muscle mass" would be an example of a mesocycle. In this 12-month program, we are going to cycle through four distinct mesocycles, each of which is designed to target one specific adaptation. They run consecutively so that when one ends, the next begins.

Each of the following 4 mesocycles should last about 3-months:

- **Wake-up Cycle:** Psychological adaptations

- **Strength Cycle:** Neurological adaptations

- **Hypertrophy Cycle:** Muscular hypertrophy

- **Cut Cycle:** Reduce body fat

Wake-up Mesocycle

- Duration: About 3 months
- Goal: To establish habits and routines that enable 80% program compliance

If you are new to working out, or if you're coming back from a break of many years, then the very first thing you should do is get your mind right. If trainees are going to quit, they do it within the first 3-months. Focusing on the psychological adaptations necessary to stick with a program for the long-haul is the crucial first step. There is simply no point in learning all this stuff if you're just going to quit. It all goes back to the KMD Dynamic. For the first few months, I see trainees struggle to get their schedules together so they can make it to the gym. They try going at 5:00 am until that doesn't work. Then they try going at night, but the wife wants help putting the kids to bed. Then they start traveling for work or football season starts or the holidays hit. New trainees struggle with all the distractions in their life. What they don't realize is that in order to make time for the gym, they have to cut other things out. Getting in shape means setting time aside for exercise, for not eating out nearly as much, for cutting alcohol, and for just generally saying no to anything that is contrary to the fitness goal. Too many guys think they can keep the exact same lifestyle and just hit the gym occasionally, and all their physique dreams will come true. This is another side-effect of dishonest fitness marketing. "Get ripped in just a few minutes a day, right from home!" If you could get a bodybuilder physique doing calisthenics at home, wouldn't top bodybuilders just do that instead of grinding for hours a day at the gym under hundreds of pounds of pig iron?

Anyway, my point being, when you first start a fitness program, there is an adjustment period. When you first start, don't worry about how much weight you lift. Worry first about actually making it to the gym on the days you're supposed to go. Baby steps. Work on being consistent. Work on following your diet plan and tracking your meals like I'm going to teach you later. Work on moving your schedule around so that fitness finds priority status in your life—equal to family and career! Yes, I said it, because you're no use to anyone if you're sick or dead. A ripped body will not happen to you accidentally when you are over 40-years-old. You have to prioritize it and work on it.

The great news is, the first few months in the gym can be some of the most productive. When you first start lifting, both strength and muscle mass increase. Muscle tone improves tremendously, making you feel tighter, stronger, and harder. Your muscles stay fuller, so they appear shapelier. Use these quick, early improvements to keep you motivated as you adopt your ever-important routine.

Workout

During this first period, most trainers will have their new trainees perform circuit training, where the trainees perform one set at one machine or station and then move to another machine or station, round-and-round, all over the gym. The point of this is to (a) allow the client to familiarize themselves with the equipment and exercises, (b) give the client a chance to get used to the schedule of showing up, and (c) lightly work their whole body and "wake it up," so to speak, without going so hard or heavy as to risk injury. I do not like circuits. I think circuits (a) cause trainees to hog the equipment, which is rude, (b) make your entire body sore those first few weeks, and (c) do not allow the trainee to spend enough time at any single exercise to really learn proper technique. Instead, I program new trainees with a classic bodybuilder-style routine called

Push-Pull-Legs (PPL)

Over the years, I have developed what I call the "Rule of 3's" to help trainees stay the course through the early days of muscle soreness. It goes like this:

1. It takes 3 weeks to get through the first phase of serious muscle soreness.

2. It takes 6 weeks to feel stronger.

3. It takes 3 months to see real change in the mirror.

4. It takes 6 months to build a consistent routine of going to the gym.

Delayed Onset Muscle Soreness (DOMS), or what I call "second-day soreness," is typically a problem when you first start lifting, but it fades over time. That's not to say that even after years of training, you can't hit a hard day in the gym and feel it for several days after. You can. But it's not like the first few weeks when every exercise makes you hurt for days after. One of the main reasons I disagree with starting new trainees on full-body circuit training is that everything is going to make them hurt, and when you make them work their whole body in their first few sessions, it makes *their whole body* hurt. Then they have to come back a day or two later and do it all over again, while they're still sore everywhere. That's not fun! Nobody wants to feel like they've been hit by a bus. Instead, by splitting their body up and working only certain muscles one day, then others the following days, a new trainee can return to the gym a day or two after a workout and lift at full capacity because they're not working the same sore muscles.

For example, a common PPL **training split** would be:

- **Monday**—Push Day: Chest, shoulders, and triceps. Example exercises: bench press, overhead press, skull crushers, etc.

- **Tuesday**—Rest.

- **Wednesday**—Leg Day: Quadriceps, hamstrings, glutes, calves. Example exercises: Squat, stiff-legged deadlift, calf raises, etc.

- **Thursday**—Rest.

- **Friday**—Pull Day: Lats, traps, rhomboids, erectors, biceps. Example exercises: Pull-ups, deadlifts, bent-over rows, barbell curls, etc.

- **Saturday**—Rest.

- **Sunday**—Rest.

The upper body is worked on Monday and Friday with two rest days and a leg day in-between. That means your upper body has plenty of time to heal before you strain it again. You only hit each muscle group once per week, so when it's time to do curls or squats again, those muscles are well recuperated. This is a less-traumatic, less-discouraging, and more productive way to begin training than the typical full-body circuit a gym trainer is likely to give you.

Diet

The focus must be on nutrition even more than exercise during this first phase. You can't build a castle out of mud, and you can't build muscle out of cookies. You have to tackle your diet early, or your exercise progress will be very disappointing.

Here's a takeaway:

It is far easier and faster to lose fat than it is to gain muscle.

Nutrition is where you're going to create 80% of your returns. Old fitness sayings like, "Abs are made in the kitchen, not the gym," are true. It really is all about diet—and that's a problem for a lot of men. We are so used to drinking soda and eating fast food that we think it's a necessity, maybe even something to defend and be proud of. We have been over-fed huge portions at restaurants for so long that when we see a normal-sized portion of food, it makes us panic. We are deathly afraid of feeling any hunger because we evolved that way. It's a powerful feeling, for sure. But, let me tell you, as someone who has been through many bulk-cut cycles, you can cut your calories down, and you will adjust. If it was pure horror and misery to clean up a diet, not nearly as many people would be successful at it. It's not fun, but it's not the hardest thing you've ever done. As a general rule of thumb, it should take about 3-weeks for your appetite to adjust to a reduced-calorie, nutritious diet.

Objective

Once you are compliant with your program at least 80% of the time, then you can call the Wake-up Cycle a success and move on to the next mesocycle. An example of how to estimate that compliance percentage would be to divide the number of days you went to the gym by how many total days you were supposed to go during the prior period. For myself, I count the days where I adhere to my diet and divide it by the total number of days in the period (however long I want that period to be). So, let's say that over the last two-week period, there were two weekends, and I cheated on my diet all 4 of those weekend days. Since that means I complied with the program for 10 of the past 14 days, that puts my compliance at just 71%, which is unsatisfactory. Therefore, over the next two weeks, I need to cheat less on my diet.

The so-called **80/20 Rule** is a bit of old gym wisdom that says you can do pretty well towards your goals if you stick to your program just 80% of the time, allowing yourself to cheat the other 20%. I have found this to be true, and a lot of it is psychological. Since we know building muscle takes time—years, really—then we need a plan we can stick with for the long-haul. Few people want to be fitness robots, living, breathing, and dreaming fitness all day, every day. We need cheat days. Cheat days allow us to maintain a workout program for a very long time because it's not so oppressive and monotonous. The 80/20 Rule strikes a good balance between the gym and the rest of life. It also gives us a framework to handle exceptions, such as holidays and sick kids. It's not a license to cheat, but it is a license to live life the most balanced way you can.

Once you are in that zone of routinely going to the gym and eating right, when you're no longer struggling for motivation and missing workouts every week, then, "Congratulations!" You can now move on to the next phase.

Strength Mesocycle

- Duration: About 3 months
- Goal: To increase limit strength
- Strength and **myofibrillar hypertrophy** (increase in the size of muscle fibers) are improved through high weight, low rep training (at greater than 80% of 1RM)

Especially at first, building strength involves neurological adaptations. The human nervous system responds quickly to the increased strain placed on the body by becoming more effective at firing off the motor neurons in your muscles. Yes, over time, your muscles will grow in response to lifting heavier weight. But before that, you will see your strength rise, possibly even while your bodyweight falls, depending on how much excess body fat you start with. In fact, it appears that in order for you to coax your muscles to grow larger, you must first maximize strength.

All body tissue, including muscle, must be maintained. Your body must nourish it, replace dead cells, and so on. There is a cost to your body to keep muscle. Your muscles are like different locations in a chain of stores. If some stores are not producing, you cut them back. But, if a store is really busy, you expand it to deal with the additional business. But expanding a store's floor space is expensive. Perhaps instead, you could meet some or all of your additional capacity needs by adding more check-out lines and stockers. In this way, revenue per-square-foot is increased without the need to build-out more space. Of course, at some point, if the business keeps growing, you will eventually outgrow the current space, and new construction becomes unavoidable. In the same way, once you maximize your neurological adaptations to lifting weights, then to continue to lift more requires adding more muscle tissue—the supercompensation principle.

Also, when you first start a new program, you're going to be weak. Strength is needed to perform all the exercises to come, so by performing basic barbell movements, such as the deadlift and squat, you are preparing your body for the muscle growth to come.

Workout

There is no hard line between training programs that increase strength and those that cause muscular hypertrophy. In general, however, lifting a weight that you can only lift for 3-5 reps before failure causes more neurological adaptations than lifting a weight for 10 or more reps. A traditional strength-building strategy is to perform 5 sets of the big barbell lifts—being bench press, deadlift, squat, and overhead press—using a weight you can only lift 3-5 times per set. Think about it: a weight you can only lift 5 times, and not once more (called your 5 rep max, or 5RM) is going to be a heavier weight that one you can lift 10 times (your 10RM). Be careful here: I'm not talking about picking a weight that you can lift 10 times and then only lifting it 5 times. I'm talking about picking a weight that truly challenges you, where you aren't sure you can even get it up that fourth or fifth time.

Here I'm going to advise you, as a 40+ weightlifter, to not test your 1 rep max, or 1RM, without proper in-person training and supervision. By definition, testing your 1RM means lifting the heaviest weight you think you might lift. In other words, it's pushing your body to redline—and that's where stuff breaks. Injury prevention has got to be your number one concern. Injuries mean pain—maybe even chronic, lifelong pain—time off from the gym, possibly time off from work, doctor's bills, all that. The whole point of fitness is to *improve* our bodies, not to damage them, so all of this is pointless if you end up injured. Trust me, do not attempt a 1RM lift unless your personal trainer instructs you otherwise.

Here's a take away:

> **Never attempt to lift a weight on your own that you are not confident you can lift at least 3 times (3RM).**

Diet

Increased strength cannot happen without physiological changes; that is, actual structural changes that must be supported by sufficient nutrition. In that way, this strength mesocycle represents a growth phase in the sense used in the GMC Matrix. Growth phases require a caloric surplus, so while you may have cut calories during the Wake-Up Cycle, during a Strength Cycle, you must eat in a caloric surplus. Cutting calories while trying to get stronger is a great way to end up disappointed or injured. If you do it right, however, a few months of heavy barbell training will most likely add several pounds of muscle to your frame. We will discuss how to structure a strength training phase in the chapter on weightlifting.

Objective

This phase ends whenever your strength has increased markedly, and that's up to you to judge. I advise setting a measurable strength goal—such as, to squat 225-lbs for 5 reps—and keep this cycle going until you hit it.

Sometimes this cycle ends involuntarily due to injury, such as persistent joint ache. After weeks-and-weeks of heavy lifting, don't be surprised if your joints get angry. If the aches become bothersome, just stop. Connective tissue, such as tendons and ligaments, accumulate microtrauma that need time to heal, too. Plus, inflammation, old injuries, bone spurs, and other of life's gifts can flare up under the heavy loads of powerlifting. Take a week off, get a massage, visit a chiropractor or physical therapist. Rest and recuperate and head into the next cycle, where we'll use lighter weights. Your achy body will appreciate it and grow.

Hypertrophy Mesocycle

- Duration: About 3 months
- Goal: To increase muscle size
- **Sarcoplasmic hypertrophy** (accumulation of noncontractile muscle elements such as water, glycogen, and mitochondria) is increased through high-rep, moderate-weight training

After a few months of building strength through powerlifting-style workouts, we can turn to the fun part: pumping your muscles up. The difference between a powerlifting-style workout to build strength and a bodybuilding-style workout to build muscle mass comes down to exercise selection, rep ranges, and exercise volume.

Workout

While we build skeletal muscle limit strength in the 3-5 rep range, we maximize muscular hypertrophy in the 8-12 rep range. While the former might be considered the powerlifter range, the latter is the bodybuilder range. The reasons this rep range works for building muscle are:

1. Higher reps really bring on the "gym pump," which encourages sarcoplasmic hypertrophy.

2. A single set that lasts 45-60-seconds is known to cause more hypertrophy than shorter sets due to longer **time under tension (TUT).**

3. Shorter rest breaks (30-seconds or so) between sets causes **metabolic stress**, which also supports new muscle growth.

Diet

Just like the Strength Mesocycle, a Hypertrophy Mesocycle is a growth phase as used in the GMC Matrix. The idea is, after all, to grow more muscle. For that reason, we know we must be in a caloric surplus. You simply can't construct new adaptations without building material. But at the same time, you should not just eat anything and everything just because you're trying to gain mass. There is good mass (muscle) and bad mass (excess fat). If you gain too much fat during these growth phases, you will have to cut longer and deeper in the future to get the fat off, which puts all your new muscle at risk. You hear about bodybuilders eating 10,000 kCal per day, but you need to realize a few things about numbers like that. For one, trainees who eat that much are already big guys with a lot of muscle built over many years to maintain. But more than that, they are on PEDs. If a drug-free person ate 10,000 kCal per-day, they would gain a lot of body fat. There's how much food you can eat in a day, and then there's how much food your body can actually assimilate and turn into muscle, and as we discussed earlier, that's up to your hormones, not the executive faculties of your conscious brain. From life experience and earlier sections of this book, we know that if we eat more than our body can use, then the excess gets either excreted or stored as body fat. Therefore, it's best to eat in a fairly small caloric surplus of just a few hundred calories over maintenance to support lean muscle growth without adding pounds-and-pounds of fat. Some fat accumulation is inevitable, but we don't want to get too carried away.

Objective

Stop this phase once excess body fat accumulates. How fat or lean to go can be a confusing issue. I see popular fitness authors advise guys never to let their abs vanish. They want you to stay under 10% body fat all the time. I'm here to tell you that for the average, drug-free man, that is nigh on impossible. Doubly so for guys our age. Here's how it usually goes:

1. Trainee begins the program at 30% body fat (which is just barely considered obese).

2. Over time, the trainee reduces body fat to ~10%, revealing abdominal separation.

3. The trainee is not happy with muscle mass and wants to gain more muscle.

4. The only way to gain muscle mass is to eat in a caloric surplus.

5. After a few weeks of eating at a surplus, abdominal separation is gone because the first thing the body does is try to return to its preferred set point weight and body fat level (Metabolic Inertia, from earlier).

6. However, if the trainee keeps protein intake high and follows a progressive weight training program, even as body fat returns, the body will also build new muscle.

7. This continues until body fat exceeds a comfortable level.

I advise never letting your body fat go above 20%. I would really prefer you keep it to 15%, but that depends on your particular body. Just don't let it get too out of hand, or you'll have to diet it all back off again, and long, deep cut cycles are hazardous to muscle gains.

Cut Mesocycle
- Duration: About 3 months
- Goal: To reduce body fat

The final 3-4-month phase of the year-long program is the dreaded cut cycle. This is a good time to step back and really assess your body composition. This would be the time to get a DEXA scan done, for example, because next, we're going to dissolve that fat layer to reveal the new, toned muscle beneath.

I say "dreaded" because there is no way to cut calories and not feel at least some hunger. I know the tricks to minimize it, but if you're used to eating big portions and feeling full most of the time, your first cut cycle might rock you back on your heels a bit. There are many fad diets—Keto, Intermittent Fasting, Paleo—but all effective weight loss diets work on the same principle: eating less than your body needs to function, so it is forced to draw down energy reserves stored as body fat. There's no magic to it.

Workout
If I could finally put the nail in the coffin of one outdated fitness idea, it would be the notion that you must exercise to "burn off" excess body fat. This is simply not true. We'll cover more on this in the chapter on nutrition, but in the meantime, let me put it into perspective:

Harvard University published a handy table of calories burned during 30-minutes of activity for people of 3 different weights. I have included some relevant activities below:

Gym Activities	125-pound person (kCal)	155-pound person (kCal)	185-pound person (kCal)
Weight Lifting: general	90	112	133
Calisthenics: moderate	135	167	200
Weight Lifting: vigorous	180	223	266
Bicycling, Stationary: moderate	210	260	311
Rowing, Stationary: moderate	210	260	311
Calisthenics: vigorous	240	298	355
Circuit Training: general	240	298	355
Bicycling, Stationary: vigorous	315	391	466
Training and Sport Activities			
Golf: using a cart	105	130	155
Golf: carrying clubs	165	205	244
Swimming: general	180	223	266
Basketball: playing a game	240	298	355
Bicycling: 12-13.9 mph	240	298	355
Running: 5 mph (12 min/mile)	240	298	355
Rope Jumping	300	372	444
Outdoor Activities			
Mowing Lawn: push, power	135	167	200
Chopping & splitting wood	180	223	266
Home & Daily Life Activities			
Sleeping	19	23	28
Watching TV	23	28	33
Reading: sitting	34	42	50
Playing w/kids: moderate effort	120	149	178
Heavy Cleaning:	135	167	200
Home Repair			
Paint, paper, remodel: inside	135	167	200
Carpentry: outside	180	223	266
Occupational Activities			
Light Office Work	45	56	67
Truck Driving: sitting	60	74	89
Police Officer	75	93	111
Construction, general	165	205	244

Source: https://www.health.harvard.edu/diet-and-weight-loss/Calories-burned-in-30-minutes-of-leisure-and-routine-activities

Next, let's look at a table California State University Northridge shared with common foods and their calorie content per serving:

Food	Measure	kCal
Bagels, Plain	1 Bagel	200
Beef Steak,Sirloin,Broil,Ln+Ft	3 oz	240
Beer, Regular	12 fl oz	150
Cheeseburger, 4oz Patty	1 Sandwh	525
Cheesecake	1 Piece	280
Chicken, Fried, Batter, Breast	4.9 oz	365
Chocolate Chip Cookies,Commrcl	4 Cookie	180
Cola, Regular	12 fl oz	160
Corn Chips	1 oz	155
Doughnuts, Yeast-Leavend,Glzed	1 Donut	235
Enchilada	1 Enchld	235
Eng Muffin, Egg, Cheese, Bacon	1 Sandwh	360
Gin,Rum,Vodka,Whisky 80-Proof	1.5 fl oz	95
Ice Cream, Vanlla, Regulr 11%	1 Cup	270
Macaroni And Cheese, Home Rcpe	1 Cup	430
Milk Chocolate Candy, Plain	1 oz	145
Olive Oil	1 Tbsp	125
Pizza, Cheese	1 Slice	290
Potato Chips	10 Chips	105
Potatoes, Baked With Skin	1 Potato	220
Rice, White, Instant, Cooked	1 Cup	180
Shakes, Thick, Chocolate	10 oz	335
Shrimp, French Fried	3 oz	200
Spaghetti,Meatballs,Tomsa,Hmrp	1 Cup	330
White Cake W/ Wht Frstng,Comml	1 Piece	260
Wine, Table, Red	3.5 fl oz	75
Wine, Table, White	3.5 fl oz	80
Yellow Cake W/ Choc Frst,Frmix	1 Piece	235
Yogurt, W/ Lofat Milk,Fruitflv	8 oz	230

Source:USDA Nutrient Database for Standard Reference, Release 12,
www.nal.usda.gov/fnic/foodcomp

49

So, according to Harvard's research, a 185-lb person who performs 1-hour of weightlifting can expect to burn 266-532 kCal depending on how hard they work. I just assume my workouts burn 300 kCal per session. That's probably a low estimate as I weigh more than 185-lbs, and my workouts are intense and more like one-and-a-half hours. But still, I'd rather under-estimate calories burned than over-estimate. Why? Because as you see from the food chart above, burning 300 kCal is nothing compared to the food we eat. Just one slice of cheese pizza is almost 300 kCal. A small cheeseburger has over 500 kCal. If I go to the gym and work my butt off for an hour, I mean absolutely crush it, burning maybe 500 kCal, and then stop at McDonald's for a Quarter Pounder with cheese, medium Coca-Cola, and medium French fries—a meal that contains 1,050 kCal—then my net caloric burn for the night is a positive 550 kCal. In other words, the hardest day in the gym only burns about half the calories of a typical fast-food meal. If I want to avoid being stuck in neutral (i.e. working hard but looking the same), I have got to make sure I am not eating more calories than I need to function, and it is very easy to overeat. I'd rather err on the side of caution than assume I am not overeating when, in fact, I am.

Here's a takeaway:

> **It's better to have never eaten the calories in the first place than to burn them off in the gym later.**

I wish this point was more widely known and understood. Just yesterday, I was talking to a lady at the grocery store about fitness, and she told me, "My trainer said I could eat whatever I want as long as I exercise." That is shockingly bad, arguably unethical advice. (Is it a deceptive way to keep trainees stuck at neutral and thus coming back for training sessions forever?) We are highly evolved, tremendously efficient systems. We can do a lot of work with very little fuel. Simply put, you can easily out-eat your workout program. Worse yet, exercise can make you even more hungry than normal, causing you to eat even more. Do not count on exercise to burn calories. It's a highly inefficient approach.

Not just inefficient, but damaging to your gains. Remember, we must recover from every workout. While to your conscious mind, post-exercise soreness is just some unpleasant sensation that will go away in time, within your body, at the cellular level, that soreness represents microscopic tears and inflammation that must be healed by the mechanical activities of your cells. The reason it takes time for the soreness to pass is it takes time for the repairs to be made. Supercompensation likely does not even occur until 72-hours after a workout. When you exercise for weight loss, you burn more calories, yes, but you also cause damage to your body tissues that must be healed—except now you're in a caloric deficit, so there's less raw building material to go around. This is not a problem when you merely diet for weight loss because eating less isn't a strenuous physical activity from which you must heal. If, while eating in a caloric deficit, you increase exercise too much, you will eventually find yourself depleted, over-trained, and losing muscle. Just like during a bulk phase, you want to find a workout/rest/nutrition balance that supports strength and muscle growth without adding too much excess body fat; you don't want to over-do your cut phase to the point that you diet away your hard-earned muscle.

When you're in a cut phase, you can't expect to add muscle ("You can't build something out of nothing!"). All you're trying to accomplish is:

1. Encouraging your body to hang onto the muscle you already have; and

2. Expending more energy than you're eating so your body supplements by burning body fat.

Your workouts should still be centered around lifting weights, but feel free to lower your weights and increase reps. Add 30-60 minutes of cardio twice-per-week, and that's about as much as a drug-free trainee should do because eating reduced calories equals reduced recovery capacity and increased risk of injury. You can keep the workouts hard and possibly even increase the caloric burn by increasing exercise volume (reps times sets) and shortening rest breaks, but you must always stay vigilant against over-training.

Diet

We're going to talk more about eating for fat loss in the chapter on nutrition, but by now you get the idea: you have to eat fewer calories. This might cause you to feel hungry. But hunger is something we can deal with. After all, I said you must eat less *calories*, not necessarily less *food*.

Here are the 3 best ways to mitigate hunger pains:

1. Eat more vegetables

2. Drink more water

3. Stay busy

Hunger is a complicated beast. Sometimes we get hungry because we need sustenance: our stomachs are empty. Sometimes we get hungry because we're bored. Sometimes we get hungry because we're exposed to effective food advertising. Ultimately, the feeling of hunger is caused by the release of certain hormones. Our body releases them *in anticipation* of eating—and just about anything can cause that sense of anticipation. Thankfully, the solution for hunger, no matter what causes it, is simple: eat something! Our bodies shut off hunger hormones when they sense our stomachs are full. That's why weight loss surgeries, such as lap band, work. Shrink the stomach, and the patient can't cram as much food in, they get full faster, and the hunger stops. Fullness is a function of the *volume* of the food you eat, not the caloric density of it. In other words, a belly full of lettuce is just as filling as a belly full of cake—but at a fraction of the calories. The human stomach stretches to hold about 1-liter of contents. 1-liter of lettuce contains about 21 kCal. On the other hand, 1-liter of spaghetti and meatballs is about 1,400 kCal. Both cause the same sense of fullness and satiation, but if you ate only lettuce, you would lose weight rapidly, while if you ate only spaghetti, you would certainly gain it. In this way, by eating low-calorie, fibrous foods, and drinking a lot of water, we can keep our stomachs physically full between meals while actually losing body weight.

Here's a takeaway:

> **During a cut phase, increase the volume of green vegetables you eat and water you drink to stay full.**

That said, sitting around watching tv and thinking about food cravings and your growling stomach is not a winning strategy. Eventually, you will cave and cheat. Keeping your mind occupied thinking about things other than eating is key to success during a cut. Pick up a new hobby, paint your house, redo your flower beds, finally finish building your project car. The more active and distracted you are, the faster the days go by, and the faster the pounds come off.

Objective

A cut cycle ends when one of the following conditions is met:

- The goal body fat percentage is achieved
- A weight-loss plateau has been reached
- Trainee's goals change
- Trainee experiences **diet fatigue**

Any one of the above is a valid reason to stop a cut phase—including just because you're tired of it. There is no aspect of this system that is not meant to be cycled. If you get tired of one cycle, switch to the next. There's no need to torture yourself. What happens is trainees cut for several months until eventually, further weight loss seems unattainable (Metabolic Inertia), or they decide they want to build more muscle or strength for a while instead. Few people can start from a high-body fat, untrained state and proceed in an unwavering path directly to washboard abs. For the majority of trainees, it takes several bulks and cuts to really dial it in—and that's fine. When the cut phase has run its course, switch back to a growth cycle; that is, either a Strength Mesocycle or a Hypertrophy Mesocycle.

The following chart lays out the essential aspects of each mesocycle in this program:

MESOCYCLES

WAKE-UP CYCLE

General:
- Starting or returning
- Psychological adaptations
- Build routine
- PPL
- Unilateral dumbbell work
- Corrective work

Nutrition:
- Clean up diet
- Typically, in a caloric deficit, but can be a surplus depending on individual

Metrics:
- Commitment

STRENGTH CYCLE

General:
- Powerlifting
- Build foundation of limit strength
- Bilateral barbell work
- Mix 5x5s and 3x5s, with PPL and deload weeks
- Linear periodization

Nutrition:
- Caloric surplus

Metrics:
- Minimum 80% compliance with program
- Increased strength
- Increased fitness knowledge
- Deepened commitment
- **Try to keep body fat below 15-20%**

HYPERTROPHY CYCLE

General:
- Bodybuilding
- Muscle size (hypertrophy)
- Mix PPL with 3x5s and deload weeks
- Drop sets, Rest/Pause, Pyramid, Pre-exhaustion, Eccentrics
- Analyze and improve imbalances

Nutrition:
- Caloric surplus

Metrics:
- Minimum 80% compliance with program
- Increased aesthetics
- Increased strength
- Increased fitness knowledge
- **Try to keep body fat below 15-20%**

CUT CYCLE

General:
- Bodybuilding
- Reduce body fat
- Improve muscle definition
- Mix PPL with HITT, LISS, and deload weeks
- Short rest breaks, lighter weight

Nutrition:
- Caloric deficit
- No restaurant food
- Count Calories

Metrics:
- 95%+ compliance with program
- Increased aesthetics
- **10-12% body fat**

1 Mesocycle

~ 3 months

1 Macrocycle

~ 12 months

Microcycles
- Duration: About 1-6 weeks
- Goal: To allow time for both intense activity and recuperation

At the lowest level of any periodization scheme is the microcycle. While a macrocycle is a year or more long, and mesocycles are several months long, microcycles are typically a few days or weeks long.

For this program, I identify two significant microcycles. They are:

Working Cycles
- Duration: 4-6 weeks
- Goal: Stimulate muscular adaptations through supercompensation

A working cycle is just a normal period of hitting the gym on schedule. There are rest days during a working cycle, of course. For example, during a standard, 7-day PPL training split, there are 4 rest days. But the purpose of working cycles is to push yourself and really strive to break new records on weight lifted and volume of work.

Rest and Deload Cycles
- Duration: 1-2 weeks
- Goal: Allow our bodies to heal and grow

We do not grow in the gym. We grow while we rest. You need to get sufficient rest, and sometimes that means taking multiple days off.

A deload day is "trainer-speak" for an easy or lightweight day. A typical deload day means lowering the weight on the bar, reducing volume, or both. It's meant to be a form of **active recovery**, where you move your sore muscles through their full **ranges of motion (ROM)** but with less strain and effort than you would during a working cycle. This actually helps the muscles and connective tissue to heal more quickly, sort of like a massage.

A true **rest period**, on the other hand, means taking a week off from the gym. It's not something to worry about early in your program when you're trying to build consistency. But in time, accumulated aches and pains will probably necessitate a few extra days off, and that's fine. I recommend taking a week off from the gym every 2-months or so depending on how you feel. If you're smart about time management, you'll schedule your rest weeks on days when you know you have other activities that will keep you from the gym anyway, such as holidays, vacations, and work trips. One of the best times to take a week off is at the end of one mesocycle, right before beginning the next. Switching from a lower intensity cut phase to a higher intensity growth phase can require a few days of mental preparation as well as diet adjustment. You may also need time to visit the grocery store and stock up on food or supplements to support the coming bulk phase.

4-8-weeks of steadily going to the gym intermixed with a few deload days and a week off, especially in-between macrocycles, is a great way to strike a pace that is sustainable for the long haul.

Essential Takeaways

- Reduce calories, intensity, and volume during a cut.

- You can increase cardio during a cut, but be careful not to over-train.

- Once your weight loss plateaus, gradually switch to a bulk cycle.

- During a bulk, increase calories, intensity, and volume.

- Cycle between strength and hypertrophy programs, back and forth, every 6-12 weeks.

- Take a deload or rest week between cycles.

Chapter 5

NUTRITION

Nutrition Essentials

There is so much confusion over nutrition that I end up spending weeks trying to de-program people from all the fad diet marketing out there. It's difficult because the diets are not outright lies. If you go from pounding sodas and potato chips to follow just about any well-known diet plan, you will probably lose weight and feel better. This is due to eating fewer calories and processed foods, especially those containing refined sugar. Eating fewer calories equals weight loss, regardless of how you accomplish it.

As I continuously reiterate, we are a holistic system, and without proper nutrition, any fitness gains you might obtain from exercise will be minimal. The old adage that fitness is 80% diet is right. I think of it like this: Diet is like the gearshift in your car. You're either in forward or reverse (a caloric surplus or deficit). Exercise is like an accelerator. The harder you mash it, the faster you'll get wherever you're heading—unless you over-do it and run out of gas along the way.

But food is more than fuel and more than building material for tissue. We don't just eat for mechanical reasons. We eat for pleasure, for a celebration, because we're bored or sad or feeling tired. There is a huge psychological component to eating, and if we ignore that and pretend that we're robots, we will fail in our nutrition goals. As with this entire system, it's important to cycle and take breaks.

Nevertheless, we are just biological machines, so a basic understanding of nutrition is essential to success in the gym. Once you understand your metabolism, you will be able to joystick your body weight up and down at will. It's really all quite logical, actually. If you eat more calories than your body needs to function, you will gain weight. If you eat less, you will lose it. But let's dig deeper into that.

Total Daily Energy Expenditure (TDEE)

How many calories do you need to get through the day? Well, that depends on a few things, like how much you weigh and how active you are. The total of all the calories your body consumes in a day for all of its activities is called **Total Daily Energy Expenditure (TDEE)**. This number can be estimated fairly accurately using online calculators, such as the one at:

https://tdeecalculator.net/

If you visit that website, you will see there are several fields to complete, such as gender, age, height, and weight. Enter the correct data for you. The next field is for activity level, and this is a bit subjective. It matters how active you are during the day. An ER nurse, construction worker, ranch hand, or other person who is physically active all day burns a lot more calories than someone who works at a desk. Also, in my experience, exercise is generally trivial for the purpose of estimating activity level, so even though it may tell you to choose your activity level based on how much you exercise, I would only look at how active you are at work. If you work an office job in the "Activity" field, simply select "Sedentary." Only pick a higher activity level if you are very active throughout the day, all week long.

Once you click the "Calculate" button, the site will present your estimated maintenance calorie level. That's the number of calories needed each day to maintain your current weight, given your current activity level.

You may also notice that the calculator breaks down just how TDEE is calculated. There are 3 components to TDEE. They are **basal metabolic rate (BMR)**, **thermic effect of feeding (TEF)**, and **thermic effect of activity (TEA)**.

Basal Metabolic Rate (BMR)

Most of the energy you consume through food is used to power the all-day, every-day, involuntary bodily functions that keep you alive, such as your digestion, heartbeat, brain function, kidney function, and so on. These activities must continue even while you're asleep, or you will die. This is called your Basal Metabolic Rate (BMR), and it accounts for about 70% of TDEE. My BMR right now is about 1,940 kCal per-day. That's important to note because think of this: What would happen if I ate less than that? Would I die, since my body has less fuel than it needs just to stay alive? No, because my body can supplement its needs by pulling energy from fat stores. In other words, if I ate less than about 1,900 kCal per day and did no exercise or perform any other activity at all, I would still lose weight. In fact, when I eat only 1,700 kCal per day, my weight drops by 2-or-more-pounds per-week and will continue to do so until my bodyweight gets so low that 1,700 kCal per-day equals my maintenance calories for that weight. Makes sense, right?

Thermic Effect of Feeding (TEF)

Interestingly, when we eat, our body must ramp-up operations to digest the food. The increased energy used during digestion is called the **Thermic Effect of Feeding (TEF)**, and it accounts for about 10% of TDEE.

Thermic Effect of Activity (TEA)

I work from home, butt parked at the computer for 10-hours a day. I also exercise intensely several hours per day. Nevertheless, if I snack at my desk, I gain weight quickly. On the other hand, I once recorded my caloric intake and body weight during a stint of hard labor, cleaning up tornado debris on a ranch. Normally, during a cut diet, I can lose 1.25-lbs per week, on average. During that 4-day period, I lost 6-lbs or 1.25-lbs per day. That's 7 times my normal rate of weight loss!

The Thermic Effect of Activity (TEA) accounts for energy used for both intentional activity (exercise) and unintentional activity (**Non-Exercise Activity Thermogenesis (NEAT)**). The combined energy burn from all physical activity represents about 20% of TDEE. Note how much less that contribution is than BMR.

TOTAL DAILY ENERGY EXPENDITURE (TDEE)

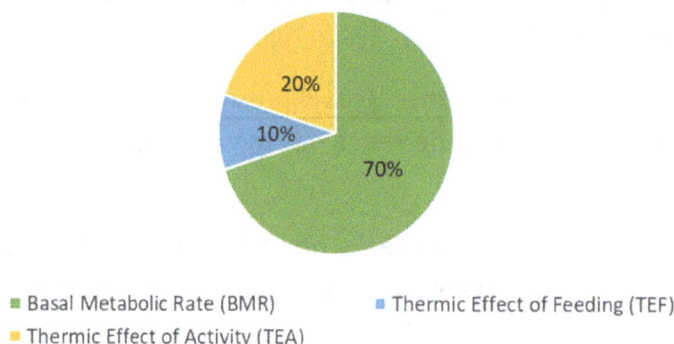

- Basal Metabolic Rate (BMR)
- Thermic Effect of Feeding (TEF)
- Thermic Effect of Activity (TEA)

Dieting for Weight Gain or Loss

As I've said before, exercising for fat loss is simply inefficient. Over-eating and then dogging yourself in the gym to burn the fat off is a recipe for disappointment and over-training syndrome. Instead, cut your caloric intake below your TDEE, and you will lose weight. The bulk of your caloric needs are to satisfy your BMR, so drop the calories and let your normal, daily bodily functions eat up your fat stores. The fewer calories you consume, the faster the weight will come off. This is what is meant by, "Abs are made in the kitchen, not the gym."

At the same time, if your goal is to gain weight (i.e., during a bulk cycle), then make it a goal to eat 500 kCal more than your TDEE. The excess calories support new tissue growth, including muscle.

Here's a takeaway:

> **To lose weight, *subtract* 500 kCal from your TDEE.**
> **To gain weight, *add* 500 kCal to your TDEE.**

In theory, this should increase or decrease your weight by 1-lb per-week. The Metabolic Inertia concept I shared earlier tells us that 500 kCal may not be enough to move the scale either direction, depending on how lean you already are, your thyroid condition, etc. If, after 2-weeks of eating at a 500 kCal surplus or deficit, your weight does not move in the desired direction, then add or subtract another 250 kCal per-day and see what happens. Keep monitoring your weight and caloric intake, and in time, you will learn exactly how many calories you need to gain or lose weight. This approach takes the guesswork out of the process and quickly puts you on a path to measurable results.

Portion Sizes

How do you know how many calories you're eating? In America, we have grown used to insane food portions, mostly driven by competition between restaurants. As a result, we have lost any idea of what a normal portion of food looks like. But we cannot trust ourselves to eat instinctively. Given a chance, humans will over-eat. I read once that the only creatures on earth that deal with obesity are humans and animals fed by humans. For that reason, when you are first learning to eat according to your fitness goals, it is a best practice to weigh, measure, and track everything you eat. You don't have to measure and track forever. If you are diligent about it, you will eventually learn how to eye-ball a proper portion of just about any food. You will also learn to recognize when you have eaten enough and when to stop. But none of this will happen instinctively because we evolved to "see food, eat food." You must consciously take measures to regulate food intake.

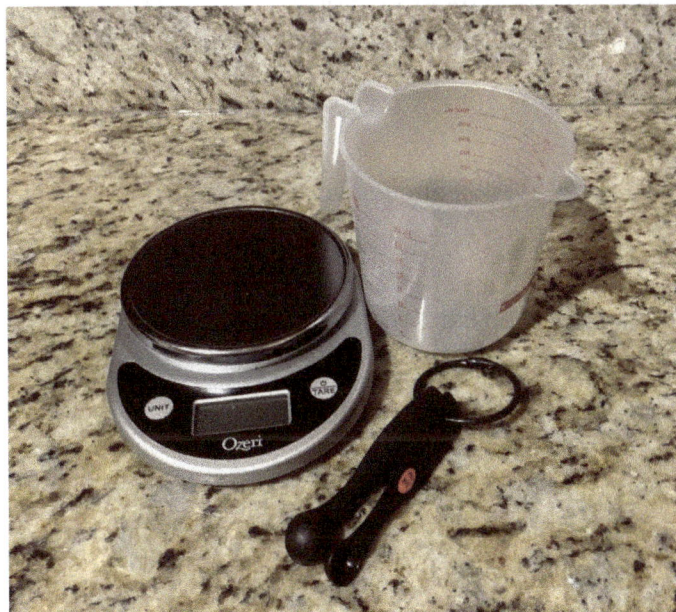

Do you know what 8 oz of chicken looks like? Can you eyeball 200 kCal of sweet potatoes? How many calories does a splash of olive oil add to a dish? Chances are, you don't know because you've always just eaten for flavor and fullness without a thought towards nutrition. Learning proper portion size requires the use of measuring spoons, a measuring cup, and a food scale. All of these items can be purchased for less than $20 total on Amazon. It takes mere seconds to weigh and measure ingredients while you're cooking. In time, you will learn to eyeball portions, and you won't need to measure anymore, but starting off, how else will you learn?

Calorie Tracking

Once you have measured your food, what do you do with that data? We need to convert food measurements into calories. How many calories are in 8 oz of chicken, anyway? Luckily, in the 21st century, there's an app for that. I have used the smartphone app MyFitnessPal for years. It's free, simple to use, and has the nutritional content of virtually every food known to man already entered. All you need to do is search for a food, enter the portion size you ate, and the app does the rest. It all gets easier over time because you will find that you eat the same things over-and-over again, and the app stores frequently eaten foods for you.

I get more resistance over tracking calories than anything else, and frankly, it's absurd. In the era of smartphone addiction, of checking social media and text messages constantly, somehow taking 2-minutes to log meals is just too much of an inconvenience.

Here's the takeaway:

Log your calories when you're sitting on the toilet.

Make this part of your daily routine. I actually pre-log everything I expect to eat that day because I already have a pretty good idea of what each meal will be. I also test out hypothetical meals to see if they fit into my daily goals.

Using MyFitnessPal

Follow these steps to set up MyFitnessPal and log your first food.

1. Go to https://tdeecalculator.net/ and calculate your TDEE.

2. Download the MyFitnessPal app from the appropriate app store for your smartphone and set up an account. The free version works fine.

3. Open the app and tap the 3 dots in the bottom right corner.

4. Scroll down to "Goals" and tap it.

5. Under goals, enter your "Current Weight." You can enter your goal weight and other things, too, if you want.

6. Under the "Nutrition Goals" section, tap on "Calorie, Carbs, Protein and Fat Goals."

7. Tap "Calories" and enter your calorie goal by adding or subtracting 500 kCal from your TDEE. MyFitnessPal will pre-enter this information based on the goals you entered earlier, but I prefer to use my own entries.

8. Next, tap on "Carbohydrates," which pops up spinners for Carbs, Protein, and Fat. We'll cover the significance of these macronutrients below, but for now, just adjust the spinners until they say Carbs = 30%, Protein = 40%, and Fat = 30%.

9. Tap the checkmark in the top right corner of the macro spinner screen.

10. Tap the back arrow in the top left corner.

11. Tap the back arrow again.

12. At the bottom of the screen, tap the big blue plus sign.

13. In the pop-ups, select "Food."

14. Select which meal you wish to enter.

15. On the resulting screen, enter the food you want to log in to the search field.

16. Once you find the food in the search results, select it.

17. Tap "Serving Size" and select the unit of measure that you're using.

18. Tap the checkmark in the top right corner to confirm.

19. Tap "Number of Servings" and enter the amount you measured using the food scale, measuring cup, or measuring spoon.

20. Tap the checkmark in the top right corner to confirm.

21. Again, tap the checkmark in the top right corner to confirm.

22. You will see the food added to your meal.

23. To add more food and more meals, tap "Add Food" on that day's meal log screen (aka the "Diary" screen).

24. You can scroll down to the bottom of the screen and tap "Nutrition" to see how your nutrients and calories are adding up for the day. You will probably find that it is easy to over-eat fat and carbs and under-eat protein.

I eat the exact same breakfast every day, so I already have that meal saved in the app. To save a frequently eaten meal, follow these steps:

1. Tap "Edit" in the top left corner of the "Diary" screen

2. Check the foods you want to include in the meal

3. Tap "Save Meal" in the bottom right corner

4. Tap "Name Your Meal" and type a name

5. Tap "Save" in the top right corner

My lunch and dinner are very similar from day-to-day, so it's not that difficult for me to open the app, decide what I'm going to eat the rest of the day, and just go ahead and pre-log all my meals. Of course, it only works if I actually eat what I say I'm going to eat.

That said, counting calories is not 100% accurate. It is much more accurate for single-ingredient foods than complicated, processed foods. For example, we're pretty sure how many calories are in an apple, but not so much an apple pie because we don't know the exact ingredients used to make the pie. There are thousands-and-thousands of different foods in most grocery stores, and while nutrition labels are instructive, they cannot be taken as gospel because most of their calories are estimated based on ingredients. Not every food was actually tested in a bomb calorimeter. Nevertheless, if you log your food and body weight, you will learn over time, in a scientifically accurate way, exactly how much energy your body needs to function. This knowledge is crucial to achieving your body composition goals, so I strongly encourage you not to skip calorie tracking.

I compare calorie tracking to budget tracking. If we don't track our spending, what happens? We overspend virtually every time. Why? Because buying stuff feels good, and we evolved to like good feelings (caused by the hormones serotonin, dopamine, and oxytocin) so our brains trick us into thinking everything is going fine. Our ancestors knew nothing but scarcity, so we evolved to eat as much as we can, whenever we can because the next meal isn't guaranteed. Our bodies produce hormones that cause food-seeking behavior, but in the modern West, scarcity isn't really a problem. (When you find yourself making a late-night ice cream run, just thank your ancestors.) The idea that we must consciously regulate our food intake rather than running on auto-pilot is the reason this book has "Executive" in the title.

- **Executive:** having the power to put plans, actions, or laws into effect.

Executive means decision-maker. It means someone who can put a plan into action. It means saying yes, but also saying no. You can either control your eating, or it will control you.

Macronutrients

There's been a lot of talk about macronutrients, or **"macros"**, in the news for years now, so everyone is familiar with the terms **protein**, **fats**, and **carbohydrates**, or **"carbs,"** but few people seem to understand their actual significance. There's this vague idea that carbs make you fat, but fat is OK now, right? Or is it not? What about saturated fat? And protein is important for some reason, right? But how much should I eat? It's actually not a simple subject, but we can reduce it all into just a few rules to follow. First, let's briefly cover the 3 macronutrients.

Protein

This is the most important macronutrient for our purposes. Protein provides the building blocks for muscle, but is the hardest macro to eat enough of. If you want to build new muscle, you need sufficient protein. You should intentionally prioritize eating protein sources, such as chicken, fish, beef, turkey, eggs, milk, and legumes.

Each gram of pure protein contains 4 kCal of energy. But didn't I just say protein is used to build tissue? Is it also used for energy? In a word, yes. Your body can use any of the macronutrients to synthesize **adenosine triphosphate (ATP)**, which is the actual energy molecule our bodies use for energy. Remember how I said earlier that if you under-feed your body and perform strenuous exercise, it may scavenge protein from your existing muscles to burn as fuel? Our bodies are miracles of adaptability.

As a general rule, you want to consume at least 1.0g of protein per pound of bodyweight. This can be increased, but the Law of Diminishing Returns comes into play as your body can only convert so much of it into muscle tissue at a time, and overeating simply leads to body fat accumulation. Plus, protein inevitably brings fat along with it, so you have to really pay attention. The best ways I have learned to hit my protein goals without also racking up a bunch of calories from fat are to:

1. Eat lean meat like top sirloin and skinless chicken breasts.

2. Supplement with whey and casein protein shakes (which we'll cover in the section on supplements).

Fat

Our bodies constantly burn a mix of macronutrients for fuel. The preferred fuel source during rest and times of low activity is dietary fat. As the intensity of activity increases, the fuel mix shifts more towards carbohydrates. This is because the cellular process that converts fat to ATP is relatively slow compared to the one that processes carbs. So, when you're sitting at your desk typing, you're running on about an 80/20 fat-to-carbs fuel mix. This is also true for **low intensity, steady-state cardio (LISS)**, such as walking on a treadmill. But when you crank the intensity up by running sprints or lifting weights, the fuel mix flips to mostly carbs.

Fats are also essential for hormone production, which, as a 40+ powerbuilder, is crucial. We need all the testosterone we can get, so cutting fat out would be detrimental to our objective.

A gram of pure fat contains 9 kCal of energy—more than twice the calories of protein. This is significant because how does fat come into our diet? By eating animal products. When we eat meat or drink milk to get protein, some dietary fat comes along with it. In fact, the fat content is what adds the most to the caloric content of the food. For example, while an 8-oz sirloin steak has 552 kCal (61g of protein and 32g of fat), an 8-oz ribeye has 614.3 kCal (56.3g of protein and 43g of fat). Ounce-for-ounce, sirloin is leaner (i.e., has more protein and less fat) than ribeye, and because fat is more caloric than protein, the sirloin has less total calories. That's why you'll hear nutritionists encourage the consumption of lean cuts of meat over fatty cuts.

There are different kinds of fats (saturated and unsaturated and all that). We're not going to get into that kind of detail here. Just know that you need a variety of fats to function optimally, so instead of stressing over the differences between monounsaturated fats and polyunsaturated fats, focus on your total calories for the day, and you will find yourself avoiding excess dietary fat, anyway. If you don't monitor fat consumption, you will find yourself eating too many calories.

I saw a guy in some documentary or another claim that all protein originally comes from plants, and that cows are merely an intermediary between us and the protein that is already in the grass they eat. Worse yet, according to the speaker, cows are inefficient in converting plant protein into animal protein, losing nearly half the grass's original protein in the muscle-building process. This is an interesting assertion. Under my theory of humans as not-that-evolved from our ancestors, I can't help but wonder why evolution left us with a taste for grilled animal fat but not grass? Everyone craves bacon and greasy French fries, but nobody has ever had a lettuce addiction.

Beware of these cravings, though. While they helped keep our ancestors alive, in the 21st century, they can cause us to overeat.

Carbohydrates

Finally, we get to the devil macro, the most hated, the most misunderstood substance in all nutrition: carbs. Carbs are much maligned in the popular fitness media these days. Why? Because we crave them, just like fats. It's evolutionary. Since we crave them, we over-eat them, and it makes us fat.

But carbs are the human body's preferred fuel source for intense activity. When you're lifting weights, you are burning glucose or blood sugar. They are also our central nervous system's (CNS) preferred fuel source. Since the brain has no fuel stores of its own, it requires a steady supply of about 120g of glucose per-day to function properly. We evolved to use carbs; we just need to be smart about how we eat them because now we are surrounded by unnatural, sugary foods that cause mayhem in our bodies.

There are two general types of carbs: simple carbs and complex carbs. Simple carbs are sugars, such as table sugar (sucrose), fruit sugar (fructose), and blood sugar (glucose). Sugars are simple molecules that can be easily digested and quickly absorbed. When we absorb a great deal of sugar at once, it causes an anabolic hormone called **insulin** to spike. Insulin's job is to tell cells to either store blood sugar or release it for fuel. When we eat a lot of sugar at once, our body immediately wants to capture it and store it as fat. This is mainly a problem with refined sugar (sucrose). Refined sugar is an unnatural substance that we did not evolve to eat. Sugar is made by plants, such as fruit, sugar beets, sugar cane, corn, etc. In its natural form, sugar is always paired with the plant's natural fiber (which is itself an indigestible carbohydrate). The fiber helps to slow the sugar's absorption into your system, reducing your body's insulin response. This is what is meant by low glycemic index (GI) food versus high GI food. Low GI food absorbs more slowly and causes less of an insulin spike than high GI food. People who are diagnosed with insulin resistance and diabetes are prescribed low GI diets. There's a lesson there for all of us. Insulin resistance and Type 2 diabetes are caused by poor diets, such as eating too much refined sugar. For this reason, the more you can remove refined sugar from your diet, the better. It really does lead to body fat accumulation and other problems.

But what about complex carbs, or what we sometimes call starches? Complex carb molecules are long strings of sugars bound together. Because the molecules must be broken down in digestion before they can be absorbed, they do not cause as much of an insulin response. We get complex carbs from potatoes, rice, cereals like oatmeal, and whole-grain bread.

Glucose, Dextrose, and Glycogen

All dietary carbs get broken down and converted into glucose in the liver. Some of the glucose then gets fused into a complex carbohydrate called glycogen for storage. I think of glycogen as an intermediate storage format between pure glucose (quick deployment) and body fat (slow deployment). The liver keeps some of the glycogen, and the rest gets stored in your muscles for quick access during intense activity, such as lifting weights. Interestingly, glycogen stored in your muscles adds fullness to them, so bodybuilders gorge on carbs the day before a competition so their muscles will appear as full as possible. Glycogen also binds with water at a ratio of up to 4-to-1, so that 2-lbs of glycogen can retain up to 8-lbs of water, for a total of 10-lbs of stored weight that is neither muscle nor fat. When your body consumes the glycogen, the water is released. This is how people lose 10-lbs in the first few days or weeks of starting a new diet or workout program: they consume their glycogen stores, causing the water weight to flush out.

Your body depletes its glycogen stores when you lift weights, which leaves your body starved for glucose as it wants to replace those stores. Within 45 minutes of completing a workout and especially during a bulk cycle, it is important that you consume simple carbs. That narrow window is the *only* time that I will recommend eating sugar. The best source of simple carbs to replenish glycogen stores is a cheap sugar extracted from corn called **dextrose** or **maltodextrin**. That's because dextrose is chemically equivalent to glucose, which is blood sugar. Your body can absorb dextrose as quickly and easily as pure glucose, and the resulting insulin response tells your cells to store it as glycogen. This is important because if you run low on glucose, the next sources your body looks to synthesize glucose from is protein, which it could scavenge from your existing muscle tissue. In this way, consuming dextrose after your workout actually protects your muscles and replenishes your energy stores for the next session.

Every day before I go to the gym, I prepare a post-workout supplement shake. I put a scoop of whey protein, a scoop of creatine, a scoop of dextrose in a shaker, and throw it in my gym bag. As soon as I'm done working out, I dump my water bottle into the shaker, shake it up, and drink it on the drive home. If I'm on a cut and a full scoop of dextrose doesn't fit into my macros or calorie allotments for the day, I use half a scoop.

Here's the takeaway:

Put a scoop (or half a scoop) of dextrose in your post-workout shake and drink it immediately after your workout.

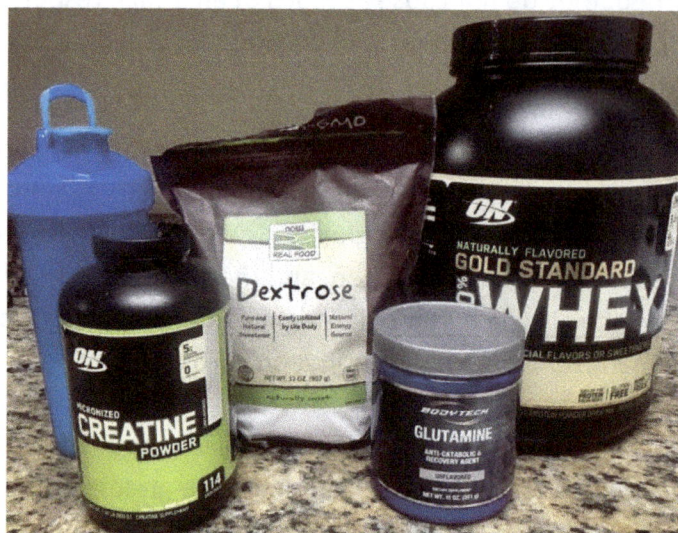

A gram of pure carbohydrates provides 4 kCal of energy, the same as protein, and less than half the calories of fat. We need carbs for proper brain function, and if we don't eat them, our body will make glucose out of protein, anyway. Carbs are our go-to fuel for lifting weights, and increasing carbs is an important part of a bulk phase. So why are carbs the devil nowadays? Because food manufacturers started putting refined sugar into everything we eat, and we have not evolved to eat refined sugar, which is a huge health problem. Refined sugar causes havoc in our systems, resulting in obesity, insulin resistance, diabetes, and, frankly, death. A small amount of sugar won't kill you, obviously. But you should make every effort to reduce your consumption of refined sugars. Soda, candy, cookies, and other sweets must be strictly rationed, and if you want to see <10% body fat, you should plan on eliminating them altogether. People with abs do not drink sodas and eat ice cream, I assure you.

40/30/30 Macro Split

You should always eat a balanced diet that includes fat, protein, and carbs. But exactly how much of each should you eat? That really differs from person-to-person, based a lot on what your lifestyle is like. If your job is physically demanding, you will need more carbs for energy. If you work at a desk, you will still need some carbs for that all-important brain function and to power your gym sessions, but you won't need as much. In general, you don't want to eat a single gram of carbs more than you need, but figuring out your particular needs takes a little trial-and-error. I start everyone with a basic split, with 40% of calories come from protein, 30% from fat, and 30% from carbs. Remember the macronutrient spinners in MyFitnessPal? This is where you would set those.

The 40/30/30 split tilts slightly in favor of protein. Start there. If, after a few weeks of at least 80% compliance with the plan, you find yourself fatigued at the gym or work, increase your carb intake by 5% and drop the fat spinner by 5%. If that still doesn't work, try adding some more carbs and 100-200 more calories per-day. You may be under-eating, over-training, under-resting, stressed, nursing a bug, have low testosterone, or any number of things, so don't just start pounding birthday cake thinking it's going to fix your fatigue. Take a gradual approach and look at all possible factors first.

Also, if you're on a bulk, eat more carbs. If your fat loss is stuck, try cutting carbs, but don't go below 100g per day (unless your personal trainer OK's it). Fat comes along with protein, and since it's the most calorically dense macronutrient, eating excess fat can cause you to exceed your target calories for the day pretty easily. Keep an eye on it in MyFitnessPal. Sometimes, I'll eat one big steak, and my daily fat intake will shoot from 30% to 60% of my daily caloric intake. The hardest thing you may face is eating 1.0g of protein per pound of body weight while also hitting your other calorie and macronutrient goals. All I can say is, I design nutrition plans based on these parameters all the time, so it is doable. I will show you an example 40/30/30 meal plan at the end to demonstrate.

40/30/30 MACRONUTRIENT SPLIT

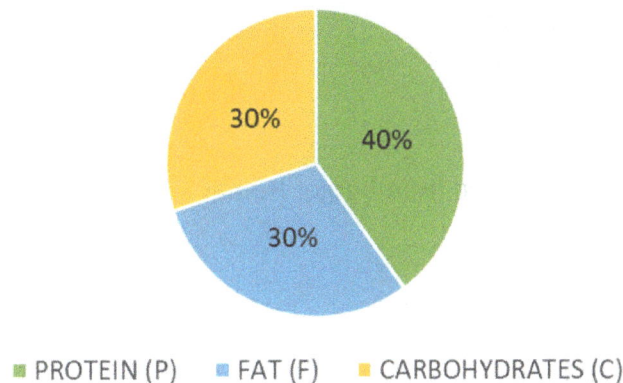

■ PROTEIN (P)　　■ FAT (F)　　■ CARBOHYDRATES (C)

Natural Foods vs. Processed Foods

A key tenet of the Monkey in a Tuxedo Theory is that our biology evolves slowly while technology evolves quickly. In less than 100 years, we have switched from eating mostly whole foods to consuming a great deal of highly processed, packaged foods made in factories—and that trend will only continue as climate change fear drives more food innovations. From plant-based pseudo-burgers to cultured meat (look it up), food scientists and entrepreneurs are figuring out more ways to construct food in factories and laboratories. The trouble is, the human anatomy is a vastly complex system that we still don't understand perfectly. We don't know how our bodies will react to these newly manufactured foods.

After WWII, health experts and the food industry turned against dietary fat because of studies linking saturated fats to heart disease. The trouble is, humans prefer the taste of two things over everything else: fats and sugars. When you take the fat out of natural foods through processing, you're left with a bland, unexciting product. In order to satisfy customers and stay competitive, food manufacturers began adding sugar and strange chemicals to our food. Since then, Americans have become increasingly obese. Our bodies simply do not evolve as fast as our ideas, and just because we can make a new food doesn't mean our bodies will know what to do with it. According to the Centers for Disease Control, in 1958, just 0.93% of the US population was diabetic. By 2015, that rate had increased to 7.4%—a nearly 800% increase in just 57 years. (Centers for Disease Control (2017). *Long-term Trends in Diabetes*. Retrieved from https://www.cdc.gov/diabetes/ statistics/slides/long_term_trends.pdf).

For these reasons, you should always choose the single-ingredient, natural food source over the processed mystery food.

- Examples of foods to **eat**:

  - Protein—Chicken breast, turkey, lean steak (top sirloin), fish, eggs, milk

  - Carbohydrates—Potatoes, sweet potatoes, rice, oatmeal, whole fruit

  - Fats—Accompanies protein, nuts, avocado

  - Vegetables of all colors

- Examples of foods to **avoid**:

  - Bread, pasta, boxed food (Hamburger Helper)

  - Fast food

  - Restaurant food

  - Fatty salad dressings

  - Cheese

  - Peanut butter

  - Alcohol

The Importance of Vegetables

I enjoy reading about our ancient hunter-gatherer ancestors and all the scientific research into what ancient people ate. We'll likely never know for sure what humans ate 100,000 years ago, but the best available studies now outline a theory based on archaeological digs and the diets of surviving hunter-gathering people. It turns out, they eat both meat and vegetables, but hunting is less successful than gathering, so they end up eating much more plant foods than animal foods. This is why people can survive on a vegan diet (with the supplementation of certain vitamins). We evolved to eat lots of vegetables of all kinds, shapes, and colors. We need a variety of nutrients from these plants to function properly. Chances are, you're not eating enough vegetables, and that's something you need to fix.

Here's the takeaway:

Eat a large serving or two of raw or steamed vegetables at every lunch and dinner.

How to Build a Meal

Using all the ideas discussed above, constructing a healthy meal is actually very simple. I cook virtually every meal I eat in a skillet, grill pan, or microwave. When you're cooking single-ingredient foods, you don't need a bunch of fancy equipment or recipes.

Here are the steps:

1. Start by deciding which protein you're going to have (chicken, turkey, beef, fish, eggs). Shoot for 0.8-1.5 grams of protein per pound of body weight, depending on your caloric needs.

2. Next, add the correct serving of complex carbs for your current diet phase (potatoes, rice, quinoa, oatmeal). If I'm on a cut diet, I eat all my carbs at breakfast, typically a bowl of 1-minute oatmeal with some fruit. Lunch and dinner are lean meat and vegetables only. If I'm on a bulk, on the other hand, I add complex carbs to dinner, which is the meal I eat right after the gym. The amount of carbs you add needs to be in alignment with your daily calorie and macronutrient goals, so always check MyFitnessPal before adding carbs to make sure you haven't already exceeded your allocation for the day.

3. Last, pile vegetables onto your plate until it looks like a filling meal to you. I eat a lot of bagged, pre-washed salad and those vegetable steamer bags available in the cooler section of the grocery store. They make a variety of vegetable steamer bags that can be quickly microwaved while you're grilling the meat.

Cut Diet Considerations

During a cut phase, continue to eat as much protein as possible because you need it to maintain muscle. What you want to do is reduce total energy intake, so cut carbs first, then fats, then protein last, if absolutely necessary. Don't cut carbs below 100g or so and don't go too extreme cutting fat. Keep a healthy, balanced diet; just reduce the energy side of the plate. As I said above, for me, that means eliminating carbs from most meals, though I never cut them completely from my diet.

The toughest part of cutting is avoiding snacks between meals. Everything you eat counts towards your daily calorie allowance, including snacks. You must log all your snacks into MyFitnessPal, or you will torpedo your weight loss efforts. But at the same time, if you find yourself starving, then eat! It is far better that you eat something and quiet your ravenous stomach than become so disenfranchised with your diet that you quit. Don't let hunger torture you. I have found that it takes about 3 weeks for my appetite to adjust downwards after switching from a bulk diet to a cut. If my stomach starts growling between meals and it's bothersome, I eat a snack. That simple. Who cares if I miss my calorie goal that day by a little? The 80/20 Rule protects me to an extent, and it's far better to cheat here-and-there to preserve my sanity than to fall off the wagon completely because my diet is too harsh.

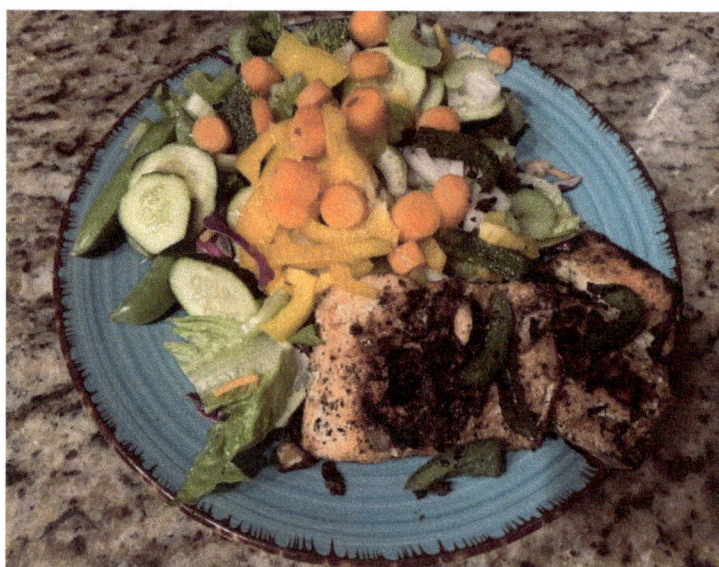

6oz of grilled salmon with green bell peppers,
garden salad, and fat-free Italian dressing

Supplements

Do you want to know the number one question new trainees ask me?

"Which supplements should I be taking?"

I bet you're not shocked. I bet some of you have asked this same question. It's truly a testament to the power of marketing that people think they have to buy all these supplements to get fit. People still think they can get steroid-like results from whey protein and creatine.

After consuming hundreds of tubs and pill bottles and eye droppers, I can assure you that supplements *might* account for 5% of gains. They are over-sold, over-promised, and many are nothing but snake oil potions. Some, like BCAAs, must be an outright lie because I have never noticed a single benefit from them. As a general rule, you can skip supplements and spend the money on real food.

But, that said, there are a few supplements that have some value. They are:

- **Fish oil capsules**: Take the recommended dose daily.

- **Multivitamins:** Take the recommended dose daily.

- **Whey protein**: A quick-absorbing milk protein. Use as much as needed to supplement whole food protein sources, especially right after exercise. I always buy vanilla whey because it mixes well with fruity pre-workout powders.

- **Casein protein**: Slow absorbing milk protein suitable for recovery while you sleep.

- **Creatine**: Add recommended dose to post-workout shake. Creatine is a natural compound already in your system that supports rapid energy recovery during exercise, allowing you to work harder in the gym.

- **Pre-workout or caffeine**: Add recommended dose to pre-workout shake, or drink a cup of coffee before hitting the gym. Cut dose in half if you feel over-amped or groggy from excess caffeine. Caffeine boosts energy and improves muscle contractions.

- **Dextrose**: Add 0.5-1.0 scoops to post-workout shake depending on calorie allowance to replenish glycogen stores and protect muscle from exercise-induced catabolism.

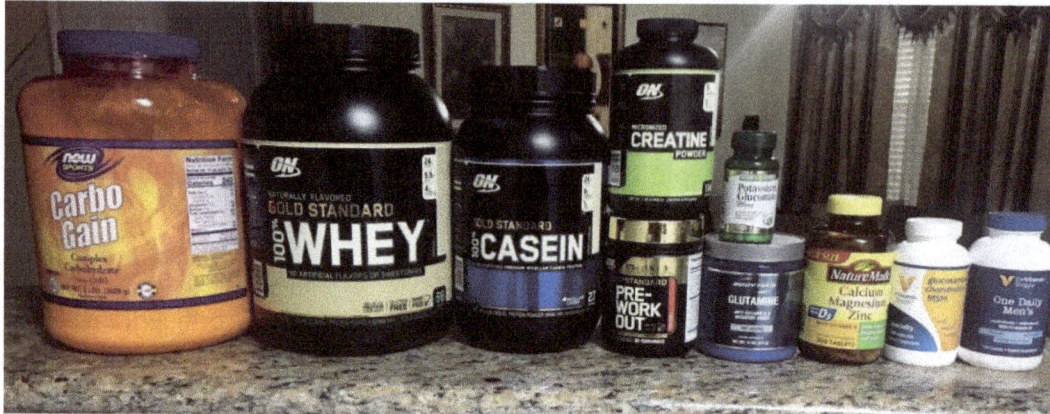

Supplement Timing and Shake Ingredients

There are 3 times per day when I recommend consuming a supplement shake:

1. **Pre-workout shake**:

   When: 1 hour before a workout

   - 1 serving pre-workout powder
   - 1 serving whey protein
   - Water

2. **Post-workout shake:**

   When: Immediately after a workout

   - 1 serving whey protein
   - 1 serving creatine
   - 1 serving dextrose (a.k.a. maltodextrin)
   - Water

3. **Pre-bedtime shake**

   When: 1 hour before bedtime. (Note that this shake may cause frequent urination at night)

   - 1 serving casein protein before bed
   - Water on a cut and milk on a bulk

Meal Timing

Some people swear by skipping breakfast or even lunch (Intermittent Fasting) or not eating after dark. You should be skeptical of anything that sounds like a hack or cheat code. Whether you eat at noon or midnight matters far less than how many calories you're eating, how many you're burning, and what those calories consist of (i.e., natural foods in the correct proportions versus a greasy sack full of fast food).

Nevertheless, due to all the confusion, let me address it quickly with a few simple ideas:

- Eat 5-6 meals per day. Supplement shakes count as meals. A typical day might consist of breakfast, lunch, dinner, a pre-workout shake, a post-workout shake, and a pre-bedtime shake.

- Snacks are ok, even if you're on a cut, but you must log them into MyFitnessPal.

Compliance

Your fitness success will be proportionate to your compliance with this program. That said, you can do pretty well at 80% consistency. Just know that 6 pack abs require 100% compliance. You may find that such an austere regime conflicts with your lifestyle. You may prefer eating out a few times a week over having abs—and that's OK. There is a lot of room for improvement when you're starting from 0. When you go from eating right 0% of the time to 80% or 50% or even 30%, that's an improvement, and you will see a return for your effort. Hopefully, in time, small improvements will motivate you to dig even deeper and boost compliance so you can reap even more rewards. You don't have to implement all of these changes at once. It's not a binary, win/lose situation. Partial improvements count along the path to ultimate victory.

Fad Diets

I can't lie. It irks me when a trainee comes to me with a head full of ideas from social media. I have people brand-new to fitness message me things like, "I've been doing intermittent fasting for a few weeks, and I'd love it if you'd help me stay consistent on it." Um, no. In fact, I can't think of anything I'd rather do less. I try to explain that "fitness" is a multi-headed hydra. There is fitness the *activity*, fitness the *business*, fitness the *competitive sport*, and fitness the *illusion*. Sorting through all this is exactly what I've been doing all these years. As a trainer, I attend not just fitness training events but also business seminars related to the field. The simple truth is that fitness training is a crowded, highly competitive field. For most trainers, making it in this industry would be a dream come true, because exercise is their passion. So, trainers are typically highly motivated to succeed in the *business* of fitness, and that means making sales. Making sales in a competitive business means either standing out—being loud and different—or riding a current trend, which is what a good deal of fitness *business* people do. All it takes is somebody grabbing onto a scientific study—no matter how dated or questionable—and turning it into the latest marketable product to set off a whole new fad. Consumers like to think they're buying the latest, greatest scientific discovery or a secret technique used only by professionals or whatever program some celebrity purportedly used to get buff. It's all driven by sales and marketing for the benefit of the fitness entrepreneur, not the trainee.

Which do you think is an easier sales pitch?

1. "Eat right and lift weights for a long time," or

2. "Eat these 3 superfoods and exercise at home for just 15-minutes a day!"

I think you get it. The *business* of fitness will always be here to sell you more supplements, more home exercise equipment, more feel-good workout programs, and more fad diets. I have given you the tools to evaluate these gimmicks and schemes on your own. A fad diet works if it puts you into a caloric deficit. There is no other trick to it. All that said, if your diet works for you, then stick with it.

Food Costs

I hear it all the time: "Healthy food is too expensive." People have convinced themselves that fast food, with all that industry's advertising expenses, is cheaper than basic vegetables and meat. I got so tired of it that I have shared numerous comparisons of meals I eat every day versus the cost of fast food combo meals.

Last year, I added up each month's grocery bill for the two adults in my household. Excluding the 4-6 times per month we eat out, our combined grocery bills averaged $626.22 per month. That number is actually high because it includes not just food but also toiletries, cleaning supplies, and an 8.25% sales tax. That means that we each eat for less than $20.00 per day or about $6.25 per meal. A medium Big Mac combo at McDonald's costs $6.48.

It takes me about 10-minutes to grill a piece of meat and either chop up a salad or steam some vegetables in the microwave. If I had to leave my home office, get in my car, drive to the nearest fast-food joint, order my food, and sit down to eat it, it would take longer than 10-minutes.

Here's the takeaway:

Cooking at home is cheaper, healthier, and more convenient than eating out.

Meal Prep

Meal prep provides all the same health, time, and financial savings that cooking at home always provides. Just buy the containers from Amazon or Walmart for a few dollars. You have options as to when and how to fill them. You could:

- Buy raw food and cook it on Sunday night so you can package it up for the entire week.

- Buy raw food and cook each meal the night before work.

- Buy pre-cooked meat to save time and package it daily or weekly.

I do a little bit of all these. I have found that pre-cooked, frozen chicken and beef fajitas are great, as well as pre-cooked brisket. I also cook a lot of pot roast and eat on it for a few days.

Another option is to buy meals from a meal prep service. Those continue to pop up everywhere. Be prepared to pay about double what it would cost for you to do it yourself, though.

Essential Takeaways

- Eat in a caloric surplus to gain weight and a deficit to lose it.

- Measure food and track calories to build good habits.

- Eat all 3 macronutrients, but cut carbs first, then fats, when trying to lose fat.

- Eat at least 1g of protein per pound of bodyweight.

- Pile on vegetables, especially to stay full during a cut.

- You don't need supplements, but they can help.

- Always choose whole, natural foods over processed and synthetic foods.

- The 80/20 rule works for the long haul.

Chapter 6

WEIGHTLIFTING

Weightlifting Essentials

What's the best deadlift technique for building strength and muscle?

a) Sumo Deadlift.

b) Romanian Deadlift.

c) Traditional Deadlift.

d) It doesn't matter which version you use. Try them all! Gains come over a long period. What matters is your overall strategy, consistency, and progressive overload. Switch exercises up to keep it fun. Exercise variety can help you stay interested in fitness for the long haul.

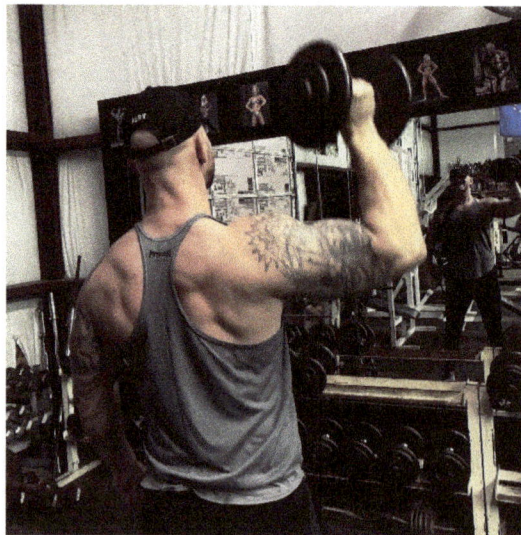

By now, you know the correct answer is "D." We're all about the Big Picture here, and which lift you perform today is less important than consistently lifting weights for months or years.

A tremendous amount gets published about **exercise selection**. Why? Because putting together unique workout programs is the best way, trainers have to differentiate themselves from other trainers in a crowded market. Plus, online training has enabled trainers to serve thousands of clients across the globe, while in the past, they were limited to working with a few clients one-on-one in their gym or home town. The best way to cash-in on the internet training boom is to sell packaged workout programs, which requires marketing, which requires being different from the competition. If I can convince you that my exercise selection and workout plan construction is better than my competitions, then you'll buy my program. Also, people don't like to think about diet too much, especially men. They would much rather think about the active part of the formula, the fun part, which is lifting weights.

I'm not saying exercise selection doesn't matter. It does matter because some exercises are less efficient than others, and some are just plain bad. But guess what? When you're first coming off the couch, lifting anything will bring results. Obsessing over which version of a deadlift to perform is silly if you're carrying 30% body fat and can't deadlift at least your body weight (using whatever technique you want). I have guys who hit the gym sporadically a few times a year trying to talk to me about a better way to perform bicep curls or something, and I can't help but tune them out. Every big, muscular guy got there by spending the great majority of his gym time performing basic lifts like the bench press, squat, and lateral raise. Once you hit plateaus on the core lifts (either physically or psychologically, i.e., if you get bored with them) or if you have an injury, you must workaround or a muscular imbalance to correct, then you can worry about obscure exercise techniques. Until then, just focus on the basic lifts, and you will get the greatest results.

Let's recap some of the weightlifting basics we've already covered:

- Progressive overload is essential to continued muscle and strength increases. There are several ways to accomplish this:

  - **Increase Intensity:** Increase the weight lifted over time

  - **Increase Volume:** Increase sets and/or reps over time

  - **Increase Density:** Decrease rest breaks between sets over time

  - **Increase Tension:** Increase the time it takes to complete each rep over time

- Strength and myofibrillar hypertrophy (increase in the size of muscle fibers) are improved through high weight, low rep training (at greater than 80% of 1RM)

- Sarcoplasmic hypertrophy (accumulation of noncontractile muscle elements such as water, glycogen, and mitochondria) is increased through high-rep, moderate-weight training

So, for strength and muscle density, we want to lift heavy weights in the 3-5 rep range, and for that pumped-up bodybuilder look, we want to lift moderate weights in the 8-12 rep range. We'll get deeper into the two different styles of training in a moment, but first, let's learn some new topics.

Warmup and Stretch

The importance of warming up and stretching for the over-40 weightlifter cannot be overstated.

If you don't thoroughly warm-up and stretch before lifting weights, you will eventually injure yourself.

Everyone agrees that you must perform a general warmup before lifting weights. But there is a body of trainers who will tell you that stretching before you lift is bad. I tested this theory, and from experience, I can assure you that's bull. In fact, the truth is the exact opposite: *not* stretching will hurt you.

Warming up doesn't have to be a big deal, and it should not tax you. The idea is to raise your core temperature. Keep a hoodie on if it's chilly. There are many ways to warm up. Personally, I've developed a routine over the years of intermixing sets of 50 jumping jacks with sets of 20 bodyweight squats because these get my temperature up quickly. In between sets, perform various stretches, all at the same time. I don't time anything, but 5 minutes is about right for a warmup. Many people prefer a light jog on the treadmill or a few minutes on an elliptical. These are great, too. Once you've got your heart going and maybe just starting to get a light sweat going—about the point, you want to take that hoodie off—you're good and warm and ready to stretch.

There are two main kinds of stretching I want you to use:

- **Static stretching**: This is the one that has fallen out of favor with other trainers, but I don't care. It's still in with me. This is the old stretching you learned in physical education class, where you bend and touch your toes and hold it, and so on. You don't have to stretch your whole body, but you can. You should at least focus on the muscles you plan to work that day, but stretching out the soreness from previous workouts can help bring some relief, too. Hold each stretch for at least 30 seconds.

- **Dynamic stretching**: This is my favorite. When you do a set of bench press or pushups, and your chest is tight, it makes you want to flap your arms front-to-back for some reason, right? You can feel it pumping the lactic acid and other waste out of your muscle, flush it with new blood, and loosen the tension in the temporarily exhausted muscles. That's dynamic stretching. Another one would be swinging your leg like you're kicking a ball. The idea is to swing your limbs through wider-and-wider arches.

Again, I can't stress enough the need to warm up and stretch thoroughly. An injury that puts you on the sideline could cost you weeks of gains, or worse. Don't ever risk an injury.

Anterior Pelvic Tilt (APT)

This is for the guys who sit behind a desk, like me. Sitting for prolonged periods of time is killing us in many ways. Did you know that when you sit, you relax your muscles, which causes all your upper-body weight to hang on your spinal column? This deadweight can put twice the normal pressure on your spine. Another thing that happens when you sit too much is your hip flexors shorten. Your hip flexors are muscles that run through your pelvis and act to tilt your pelvis forward or backward. Sitting can cause the hip flexors to shorten so that when you stand up, your lower back sways in and your butt sticks out, a postural condition called **lordosis** brought on by **anterior pelvic tilt (APT)**, meaning the top of your pelvis is tilted too far forward. You can tell if you have it if you strip down to your underwear, adjust the waistband to be comfortable on your waist, and stand sideways to the bathroom mirror. If the waistband of your underwear slopes down from front to back instead of running parallel to the floor, you likely have some lordosis going on. When you try to barbell squat, you may find that your lower back (erector spinae) muscles tighten up and hurt like hell.

The best solution I have found is a modified runner's stretch. Standing up straight, take one big step forward with your right foot into a forward lunge position. Now lean your hips forward so that you feel the front of your hip stretch on the left side where your leg is back behind you. Then, rotate your torso all the way to the left and drive your hips forward even more. Arch your back. You should feel a deep stretch at the front-left of your hip. Now switch sides and repeat. Do daily this as often as you can remember.

Reps and Sets

The action of lifting a weight one time is called **repetition** or **rep**. A group of reps performed in sequence without rest is called a **set**. The collection of all sets performed in a single training session is called a **workout**.

Every rep has two components: (1) an up, or **concentric**, portion, and (2) a down, or **eccentric,** portion. It turns out the eccentric portion is more important for gains than the concentric portion. Basically, keeping your muscles tight and controlling the weight's descent really shreds the taut muscle fibers, especially the more exhausted they are. Always make every rep count. Don't sit there and pound out a set as fast as possible, just throwing the weight around. Take your time and concentrate on form and the mind-muscle connection (which I talk about later).

I talked before about lifting for a certain number of reps to achieve specific goals—10-12 reps for hypertrophy and 3-5 reps for strength. But those are rough numbers. In reality, you should take every set to muscular failure. If you've increased weight that day on a certain lift, you may only be able to get 6-8 reps instead of 10 before the target muscles give out. By going to failure and constantly **overreaching**, you strain your body and make it grow. (Muscular fatigue is a fascinating subject in itself and beyond the scope of this book, but add it to your research topic list.)

A better strategy for executing a set would be,

> **Choose a weight you think you can lift for your target rep range and then lift it until failure. If you ended up lifting it for more reps than you thought, increase the weight.**

If I'm on a strength cycle (3-5 rep range), but I can squat the weight I chose for 8 reps before failure, then I need to increase the weight. The same is true for hypertrophy cycles. 10-12 reps are good, but if you can lift a weight for 20 reps, it's not heavy enough (unless you're rehabbing an injury).

Volume

We define exercise "volume" as:

Total sets x reps x weight lifted

Here are two examples:

Example 1: 3 sets of 10 @ 200-lbs = 3 x 10 x 200 = 6,000

Example 2: 5 sets of 5 @ 240-lbs = 5 x 5 x 240 = 6,000

Notice that while Example 1 has us performing 3 sets in the 10 rep range (which is the hypertrophy range) and Example 2 has us performing 5 sets in the 5 rep range with a heavier weight (which is the strength range), they both equal the same exercise volume. Volume matters for gains. If your exercise volume is too low, gains will be low. Then again, if volume is too high, gains will also be low. This comes into play with the concept of **Maximum Recoverable Volume (MRV)**, which we will discuss later.

Post-exhaustion Training

The following is one of the most important principles I can teach you. Your workouts will become massively more efficient and effective if you will design all your programs using post-exhaustion:

- **Post-exhaustion training:** Perform compound-joint lifts *before* single-joint lifts.

Let's break this down. What's the difference between compound-joint and single-joint exercises?

- **Single-joint exercise:** An exercise that involves movement through only one joint, also called an isolation exercise. Examples are bicep curls (movement through elbow only), calf raises (movement through ankle only), and dumbbell chest flies (movement through shoulder only).

- **Compound-joint exercise:** An exercise that involves moving through more than one joint. Examples are bench press (movement through shoulder and elbow), squats (movement through hips, knees, and ankles), and pull-ups (movement through shoulder and elbow).

Compound lifts use more muscle and therefore require more energy to complete, so you always do those first. If, for example, you performed triceps extensions first then tried to follow with bench press, you will find that your triceps—one of the weaker muscles used in the bench press— is already tired, so you won't be able to lift as much. That's a problem because the goal of the bench press is to overload the pecs (chest muscles). If you reduce the weight you can lift by pre-exhausting your triceps, then you will not be able to overload your pecs as effectively.

I may be able to barbell bench press 225-lbs, but I seriously doubt I could cable triceps extension that much. Isolation exercises use less muscle than compound exercises, and therefore you can't lift as much. Think about it. Which is better: Lifting heavy weights when you're fresh at the start of your workout, or last once you're already tired? At the same time, and to our benefit, performing compound lifts first pre-exhausts the target muscle, so when you perform single-joint lifts later in the workout, you can really focus on taking that muscle to total failure.

A few basic examples:

- On Leg Day, perform barbell squats *before* seated leg extensions or hip thrusts.

- On Push Day, perform barbell or dumbbell bench press *before* triceps extensions, dumbbell flies, cable crossovers, or overhead press.

- On Pull Day, perform pull-ups or lat pulls *before* bicep curls or straight-arm pull-downs.

Building your workouts on this principle allows you to maximize your energy by hitting the big, heavy lifts at the beginning of your workout. Then you take advantage of that pre-exhaustion of your muscles later in the workout by targeting already tired muscles with specific isolation exercises designed to really fry them. There is no more efficient way to structure a workout than this.

Here's a takeaway:

Always perform heavy, compound-joint lifts *before* lighter, single-joint lifts.

Form Over Weight

If you train with me in-person in a gym, you will find I am a stickler for form. Form is everything. Form can make light weight heavy. Form can make heavy weight useless. Form can hurt you or heal you. Respect form.

When I'm in the gym, headphones in, music cranked, all I am thinking about is proper form and pushing myself as hard as possible during that set. Form is better taught in person, but you can also teach yourself through practice.

The basic principles of good form are:

- Only move through the joints you're supposed to move through. "Freeze" every other joint by flexing the surrounding muscles. This is an isometric contraction of all non-target muscles in your body.

- Perform each rep with a full range of motion (ROM).

- Perform each rep with slow, steady deliberateness.

- Do not use momentum to bounce, jerk, or throw the weight; instead, consciously "muscle" the weight up.

- Lift the weight with explosive force, then lower it more slowly.

Heavy weight often causes the form to suffer. Therefore, perfect your form using weight in the 10-12 rep range before increasing. If you don't master form before increasing weight, you will get poor results and very likely injured. It is a misconception that big weightlifters always lift heavily. In fact, there are tons of videos of pro bodybuilders like Kai Greene doing 25-lb lateral raises for high reps and The Rock doing slow, controlled reps with a weight you or I could lift. Lifting heavy weights in itself won't get you results. Lifting *correctly* will.

Rep Cadence, Time Under Tension (TUT), and Eccentrics

It is common for trainers to use a short-hand for **rep cadence** that looks like this: 3010. The 4 digits represent the 4 components of a single rep. It breaks down like this:

> 3 – Take 3-seconds to slowly lower the weight (the eccentric portion of the lift)
>
> 0 – At the bottom, do not pause
>
> 1 – Take 1-second to forcefully lift the weight (the concentric portion of the lift)
>
> 0 – At the top, do not pause

A slower set might be denoted "4020". A faster one would be "2010".

For strength, explode the weight up with as much force as possible and control it on the way down as best you can. The explosive concentric is called **compensatory acceleration**. If used properly, you can get the same effect of lifting heavier weights with lighter, safer weights.

For hypertrophy, where weights are more manageable, take 1-second to lift the weight (concentric) and 3-seconds to lower it (eccentric). Why? Because we've learned that muscle hypertrophy is maximized when a set takes greater than 40-seconds to complete. This relates to a concept called **Time Under Tension (TUT)**. Under a 3010 rep cadence, it takes 4-seconds to complete a single rep. Therefore, if you performed 10 reps per-set, each set would take 40-seconds to complete, which satisfies the TUT requirement.

But wouldn't a 1030 rep cadence or 2020, and so on, do the same? Are 4 seconds, 4 seconds, no matter what? Actually, no. In addition to TUT, we also know that slowly controlling the weight on the way down (the eccentric portion of the lift) causes more microtrauma and more supercompensation than just dropping the weight after the concentric portion of the lift. So, to get the most out of every rep, set, and workout, you should control the weight on the way down.

Here's the takeaway:

> **Using a full ROM, muscle the weight up using only the target muscles, then control the weight down for a 3-second count.**

Range of Motion (*ROM*)

With rare exceptions, you should perform every lift through the target joint's full ROM. That means lifting the weight (whether it be a barbell, dumbbell, cable attachment, or your own body weight) all the way up and all the way down. Failing to do this can (a) shorten your muscles, and (b) lead to sub-optimal growth, because you're doing sub-optimal work. It's a question of efficiency, really. More work is done through a full ROM than a partial, causing more microtrauma per-hour spent in the gym and more metabolic stress, therefore yielding faster returns.

Here's the takeaway:

> **At the bottom of a lift, you should feel the target muscle stretch, then contract hard and flex the muscle on the way up.**

Rest breaks

Keep rest breaks as short as possible, especially during a hypertrophy or cut phase. Lifting heavy weights takes longer to recover from, so 2-minutes or so between sets is common. No matter what, you should not sit, check your phone, take photos, or chit-chat between sets. That's for noobs and slackers. Get your set, pace around to flush the lactic acid out of your muscles, and speed up recovery. Pacing between sets is also easier on your heart. As soon as you catch your second wind, get your next set. Creatine can help speed recovery between sets.

Here's the takeaway:

- **For heavy lifts, rest for less than 3 minutes between sets.**

- **For hypertrophy, rest for less than 1-minute between sets.**

Mind-Muscle Connection

A lot of trainees come to me with poor "body awareness." They don't really know where their limbs are in relation to their body, especially if the limb is out of their view. There's actually a part of the brain that controls that, which means we can improve body awareness through practice.

The mind-muscle connection is one of those things that sounds like mysticism until you feel it. Once you feel it, it's obvious. Celebrity fitness trainer Jeff Cavalier once said that if you can't flex a muscle so hard that it's uncomfortable, you lack sufficient mind-muscle connection. Once you really have the connection developed, you can pretty much make your muscles cramp at will. I'm also reminded of an Old Spice commercial featuring Terry Cruz when he appears to play musical instruments using electromyography (EMG) by flexing each muscle separately, including his pecs. ("Flame sax!") I have also seen masterful belly dancers who can isolate muscle contractions in their abdominals. The mind-muscle connection is very real, and it can be developed.

When lifting, look at the target muscle. Focus your mind on the muscle being worked. Think about what it's doing. For example, grab a fairly light dumbbell (12RM) in each hand. While standing, perform alternating dumbbell biceps curls—left arm, then right arm, then left arm, etc. When you curl the weight up, look at your biceps. Use the target muscle to lift the weight (i.e., intentionally "muscle the weight up"). Watch it flex. At peak contraction, flex and hold it for a second before lowering. Once the burn starts, use that burn as a "lighthouse for your mind." Really focus on the discomfort. In time, you will become far more familiar with your body than you ever have been before.

Another great way to build a mind-muscle connection is to flex in the mirror. Try a front double biceps pose and hold it until your biceps just start to cramp. That's fairly easy. Now try to flex your lats out (the "cobra" or "wings" flex). Some people struggle with that. What about your quadriceps (the big muscles on the front of your thighs you might use for kicking a ball)? Can you flex them while standing? What about your upper traps (the muscles at the top of your back that connect your neck and shoulders)? Get in the habit of flexing each muscle in your body one-by-one every day, starting with your calves and working up to your traps. This will help train your nervous system and give you harder contractions when you lift. The isometric strain will also make your muscles more toned and appear fuller over time.

Advanced Techniques

I love advanced techniques. This is where you get to test what you're made of, push boundaries, and hopefully break through plateaus. They can put you into an over-trained state if you do them all the time, though, so don't do that. Use them if you feel stuck at a certain weight for too long (several weeks) or if you feel particularly amped that day, but don't build your entire program on them.

I'm not going to cover them all, but some examples of advanced techniques are:

- **Drop Sets**: Best performed with cables or a rack full of dumbbells. Choose a starting weight and perform 8 reps. Set the weight down and immediately either move the pin to the next lower plate or grab the next lighter dumbbells. Do 8 more reps. Lower the weight again and repeat. If you can't keep getting 8 reps, then stop and drop the weight and keep going. Lower the weight at least 3 times (for at least 3 sets in a row). I usually go from my starting weight all the way down to the lightest weight available. Only do these once per week or so, and make sure it's the last set for that exercise. (e.g., if you're doing 3 sets of biceps curls, do your first 2 sets normally and make the last set a drop set).

- **Supersets**: Perform one set of pushing (or pulling) exercise, and then, without pause, immediately execute a set of a pulling (or pushing) exercise that opposes the motion you just made. Example: Do a set of bench press and then immediately do a set of bent-over rows. Or do a set of biceps curls and then a set of triceps extensions back-to-back. I rarely use these, but they are the core of German Volume Training, which we'll cover in a moment. If you're doing them right, they will exhaust you. They are a great way to get more work done in the gym in less time, though. It's like doubling up your workout, but that's only true if you can keep the total volume up. In other words, it's all good to shuffle your entire back workout with your chest workout if you do the same number of sets and reps and lift the same weights you would if you had performed those workouts on separate days. Keep that in mind when deciding if Super Sets are truly more efficient.

- **Compound Sets**: My personal favorite. These involve performing 2 exercises back-to-back on the same muscles. The exercises can be a compound-joint followed by a single-joint. Examples would be hitting a set of pull-ups and then immediately grabbing dumbbells and hitting a set of curls. Another would be doing a set of bench press followed immediately by a set of skull crushers. These really get your muscles pumped, and the pump is important for gains (sarcoplasmic hypertrophy).

- **Rest/Pause**: Take a set to muscular failure, then let the weight hang, but don't set it down. Take a breath or two, then get 1 or 2 more reps. These are very effective and can be used more often than other advanced techniques.

- **Heavy Eccentrics**: These are the most demanding of the advanced techniques and will require the most caution and recovery time. Heavy eccentrics involves slowly lowering a weight that you can't lift yourself. This requires a partner/spotter to help lift the weight up. Basically, the two of you lift the weight together, and then they let you have it, and you fight it on the way down. This is very effective in breaking plateaus on big compound lifts like bench press and squat and will increase muscular hypertrophy relatively quickly. That said, nothing in life is free. If they are effective, that means they cause a lot of microtrauma that must be allowed extra time to heal. At the same time, heavy eccentrics cause central nervous system exhaustion above and beyond regular weightlifting techniques. Do these sparingly (maybe once a month) and then don't work that muscle group again that week.

- **Bands**: Rubber resistance bands are everywhere right now, and I like them. I carry 2 or 3 sets in my gym bag. Without getting too technical, bands can be used to effect specific changes along the so-called **strength curve**. The idea is that some lifts get easier towards lockout (full extension), so bands can be attached to weights to counter that because the farther you stretch bands, the more difficult it gets to stretch them. An example would be the bench press. When the weight is down, 1-inch above your chest, the weight is harder to lift because your muscles are at full stretch. Your triceps are basically no help at this point. But once you push the bar up and your arms get straighter-and-straighter, the weight gets easier to push up until you reach full lockout. If you attach a rubber band to either side of the bar and then run that band under the bench (or otherwise attach it to the floor), as you push the barbell away from the floor, the band gets stretched more-and-more making lockout more-and-more difficult. Think about how they can be used for bicep curls to make the lift harder at the top, where normally it is easiest. Another way to use them is just by themselves. I sometimes attach bands to a high anchor point and perform woodchoppers for my abs and obliques, for example. Bands are cheap, and there are many ways to use them. Grab a set for your gym bag and experiment. Just don't pop yourself in the eye with a 70-lb resistance band!

- **Chains**: Chains are a cool toy that powerlifters use. Similar to bands, they affect the strength curve. Picture the bench press again. Put 225-lbs on the barbell. Now hang 70-lb chains from either side, so they barely touch the floor when the barbell is racked. Now, un-rack the bar and hold it at full extension (lockout). At this point, you should have the full 225-lb bar plus the additional 140-lbs of chains bearing down on you. Now begin lowering the bar to your chest. As the distance between the bar and the floor lessens, the chains start piling up on the floor. As the bar lowers, the weight lowers. Just like with the bands above, the load is lightest at the bottom and heaviest at the top of the lift. This is an advanced strength training technique that is used to break through "sticking points" and plateaus. You won't need this until you've maxed out all your fundamental techniques.

The Pump and the Burn

Working in the 10-12 rep range makes your muscles feel like they're going to pop, and the burning in your muscles can be searing. Lifting heavily for strength just doesn't feel that way, at least not to me. A set of 3 super heavy squats will exhaust you, but in a different, more gassed, out-of-breath way. But in bodybuilding, the pump and the burn matter. This is what really causes sarcoplasmic hypertrophy, so when you're in a hypertrophy cycle, lift for the pump and the burn. Drop sets, compound sets, and lifting until failure are great techniques for this.

Training Splits

Splitting is how you divide up your body for exercise purposes. Determining how you're going to work different body parts in conjunction with each other is crucial for maximizing rest and recovery between workouts.

I'm going to give my recommendations later, but some sample training splits are:

- **Full-body split**: Train your entire body every time you hit the gym. Circuits are commonly used. Best if you can only hit the gym twice per week.

- **Push-Pull-Legs (PPL)**: Muscles that work together synergistically are exercised together, i.e., Push Day would include chest, shoulders, and triceps.

- **Upper/Lower Split**: Upper body is worked one day; lower body is worked another day.

- **Bro Split**: Each body part has its own day, i.e., chest day, leg day, shoulder day, arm day, back day.

Strength Programs

One of the most common programs for building strength is the **5x5** ("five-by-five") program. It's very simple: For each exercise, perform 5 sets of 5 reps using your 5RM weight. The workout begins with big, compound-joint lifts followed by lighter **accessory lifts**.

Just to give you an idea, a typical 5x5 workout might look like this:

- Barbell Squat—5 sets of 5 reps
- Barbell Bench Press—5 sets of 5 reps
- Bent-over Barbell Row—5 sets of 5 reps
- Barbell Curls—3 sets of 10 reps

Another common type of strength program is called **Linear Periodization**. These programs use the basic idea that as weight (intensity) increases, the number of reps you can complete decreases. These programs are favored by competitive powerlifters as a way to boost their 1RM for competition. As weeks pass leading up to competition, volume decreases and intensity increases.

A typical linear strength program might look like this:

- Week 1—Bench press 70% of 1RM for 10 reps
- Week 2—Bench press 75% of 1RM for 8 reps
- Week 3—Bench press 80% of 1RM for 6 reps
- Week 4—Bench press 85% of 1RM for 4 reps
- Competition Day—Bench press 100% of 1RM for 1 rep

A somewhat advanced training technique called **cluster sets** can also be used. Clusters are basically sets of single rep lifts with 20-second breaks in between. As with the other strength programs outlined here, clusters should be performed with the big compound lifts. They work because you use your 3RM weight, but lift it for 5 reps. Do 3-5 sets of these for each exercise.

First, lift the weight for 1 rep, then set it down, step back and take 20 seconds to catch your breath, then repeat.
A typical cluster set for deadlifts would be:

1. Put your 3RM weight on the deadlift bar
2. Lift the weight
3. Set it back down
4. 20-second break
5. Lift the weight
6. Set it back down
7. Take 20-second break
8. Repeat for 5 reps

Hypertrophy Splits
While building strength is all about lifting progressively heavier weights, lifting for hypertrophy is about volume.

My favorite hypertrophy split is called **Push, Pull, Legs (PPL)**. PPL is, in my opinion, the most efficient training split. For hypertrophy, it's important to hit each muscle from multiple angles using several exercises. Each body part might get hit by 2-5 different exercises. A chest workout might include bench press, incline bench press, flat dumbbell flies, incline dumbbell flies, and dumbbell pullovers. Perform exercises with a variety of bar grips (narrow, shoulder-width, wide, and neutral). Try performing some standing, some sitting, use cables, barbells, dumbbells, and bodyweight. One of the reasons I love hypertrophy training is that flexibility and exercise variety are encouraged. I get bored easily, so the variety keeps me excited to return to the gym.

A sample PPL split would be:

- Monday—Chest, shoulders, and triceps
- Wednesday—Quadriceps, hamstrings, glutes, calves, lower back
- Friday—Upper back, biceps

German Volume Training (GVT), also sometimes called 10x10 training, is another popular bodybuilding split. You perform 10 sets of 10 reps of each exercise, and typically, you will use supersets to speed things up.

You only perform one exercise per body part, and you want to get the most value for your time, so you only perform compound joint movements because they recruit the most muscle fibers. Also, since you have to be able to complete 10 reps in every set, including the last set, you'll have to make sure you pick a weight you can handle all the way through, meaning you need to choose a weight lighter than your current 10RM. Use that same weight throughout the set. The first few sets may seem easy for you, but the last few will be brutal. Slow down your reps to a 4020 tempo, and you will really fry your muscles.

A sample GVT workout would be:

- 10 sets of 10 reps of bench press supersetted with 10 sets of 10 reps of seated rows.

- 10 sets of 10 reps of incline bench press supersetted with 10 sets of 10 reps of barbell curls.

Reverse Pyramid Sets

You always want to make the best use of your time in the gym. A great technique to get the most out of your PPL program is called a **reverse pyramid set**. Reverse pyramiding is based on the observation that during a single workout, with each set you perform of a given exercise, the easier it gets (until you're exhausted, of course). Do a set of curls at a certain weight, take a break, then pick the same weight up again. Feels lighter, doesn't it? This is due to a short-term neurological adaptation that provides a little help on successive sets of the same exercise. This little boost allows you to increase the weight you lift on the next set, causing even more microtrauma.

Let's say your 10RM on barbell biceps curls is 60-lbs. You could perform the following reverse pyramid set:

- 1 **warm-up set** of 10 reps at 50-lbs
- 30-seconds rest
- 1 **working set** until failure at 60-lbs
- 30-seconds rest
- 1 **challenge set** until failure at 70-lbs

The **warm-up set** will be easy, but it gets you ready for the next sets. The **working set** will be tough, but you can handle it. The **challenge set** is going to be the hardest because the weight is more than your 10RM, and you're already pre-exhausted from the previous 2 sets. Maybe you can only lift it 6 times. That's fine because that's the set that really does the work for you, pushing your muscles past their limits and causing serious microtrauma.

I take it a step further with what I call **progressive pyramiding**, which is reverse pyramiding that gets heavier over time. By really pushing yourself on the challenge sets, you'll increase your strength over time, so you need to increase the weight you lift over time, too. That's the progressive overload principle.

The following diagram demonstrates:

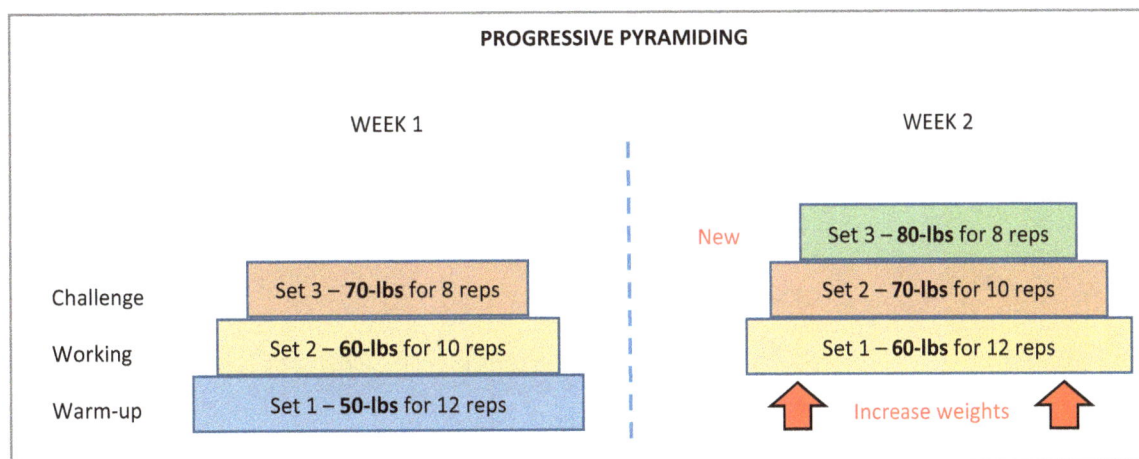

PROGRESSIVE PYRAMIDING

WEEK 1 | WEEK 2

	Week 1	Week 2
Challenge	Set 3 – **70-lbs** for 8 reps	Set 3 – **80-lbs** for 8 reps (New)
Working	Set 2 – **60-lbs** for 10 reps	Set 2 – **70-lbs** for 10 reps
Warm-up	Set 1 – **50-lbs** for 12 reps	Set 1 – **60-lbs** for 12 reps

Increase weights

Cooldown

One of the most under-appreciated elements of a solid workout program is the post-workout cooldown. Cooling down requires a few minutes of light cardio, such as walking on a treadmill. It falls into the realm of active recovery in that the point is to work the muscles gently, like a massage, to flush out all the metabolic waste from exercise and fill the muscles with fresh blood. Cooling down helps to reduce cramps and soreness. When you're done with your workout, take those extra few minutes to keep moving while you catch your breath, and your heart rate returns to normal. It helps with recovery, which is crucial for growth.

Essential Takeaways

- Always warm-up and stretch before lifting

- Cooldown afterward

- Use PPL or GVT for hypertrophy

- Use 5x5s, linear periodization, or cluster sets for strength

- Keep rest breaks as short as possible

- Form over weight

- Use post-exhaustion and progressive pyramiding

- Eccentrics matter

- Time Under Tension (TUT) matters

Chapter 7

CONDITIONING

Cardio Essentials

Nothing is more misunderstood than cardio. There are trainers who love cardio, so they program it heavily. Are they wrong? As in all things, that's not the right question. The SAID Principle says that we need to match our training with our goals. If your goal is to increase cardiovascular health, lung capacity, or burn fat, then cardio might be the right solution. If, however, your goal is to build limit strength or muscle mass, cardio is the wrong solution.

We evolved to walk and jog. We are highly efficient at those activities, burning very few calories when the effort is low. At the same time, your muscles don't need to get bigger or stronger to jog. Rather, your Type I muscle fibers and the aerobic (oxygen-based) energy system that feeds them need to get more efficient. That's why long-distance runners are not big, muscular people. Sprinters, on the other hand, often have considerable muscle development and leg strength. That's because short bouts of full-out effort do work your Type II muscle fibers and the glycolytic (glucose-based) energy system that fuels them.

Some trainees want to build muscular endurance, especially if they find themselves tiring easily, or they compete in sports. If that's the case, you need to find a careful balance between all your goals. If you're trying to build muscle *and* strength *and* endurance *and* cut fat, you are likely not going to see great results in any one of these categories. You can improve them all, yes, but it's going to take longer because some of these goals are contradictory.

The troubles with cardio for a powerbuilder are:

- You're burning calories by performing exercises that do not build muscle or strength (at least not efficiently). Therefore, you are spending time and energy on activities that do not support your primary goals.

- Cardio can cause soreness, fatigue, and injuries that can affect your weightlifting performance, especially repetitive use injuries and lower body joint pain.

- Cardio must be recovered from, so doing cardio and lifting weights can compound your fatigue.

Before performing cardio, ask yourself why you're doing it. Is it to build cardiovascular health? That could be a valid reason, especially as a man over 40. However, I would point out that intense weightlifting also causes cardiovascular strain and, therefore, improvement. If it's to burn fat, the next question is, are you in a bulk cycle or a cut cycle? Performing cardio to cut fat (i.e., lose body mass) during a bulk phase at the same time you're trying to build muscle (i.e., increase body mass) is contradictory. You're pushing and pulling at the same time. Pick one or the other.

Here's the takeaway:

- Performing cardio during a cut phase can help burn fat and even improve blood flow to your muscles through increased capillarization. But, as I've said before, you could also just eat in a caloric deficit, let your basal metabolic rate (BMR) burn the fat, and save yourself the added fatigue and recovery time.

- Performing cardio during a bulk phase is contradictory and should only be performed if your doctor insists.

There are many ways to perform cardio. Swimming, jogging, elliptical machine, stair climber machine, wind sprints, and on and on. Each of them fits into one of two types of cardio: HIIT or LISS.

HIIT – High-Intensity Interval Training
HIIT has become very popular in the last 15-years or so with entire gym franchises based on the training style opening. HIIT is what we did in wrestling practice long ago, but we called it "wind sprints." The basic idea behind HIIT is to do a bunch of exercises back-to-back at full effort. You take your body into the red zone, so to speak, and keep it there. The reasons HIIT became so popular are:

1. HIIT sessions typically don't exceed 15-minutes, meaning you can get your work done in a short time, which appeals to busy, modern people.

2. Fans of HIIT love to talk about the "afterburn effect," known by fitness pros as EPOC, or Excess Post-Exercise Oxygen Consumption. The idea is that you go so hard during the workout that you actually use more oxygen than you can breathe in, thus creating an oxygen deficit that must be paid back. Therefore, you breathe extra hard for hours after a HIIT session, which means your body continues to work a little more than normal even after the workout is complete.

While both of these points have some merit, a couple of observations of my own:

1. Most people do not perform HIIT with enough intensity to fully enjoy the benefits, taking long rest breaks between sets, and just generally don't overreach enough. If you're just doing 15-minutes of low-effort work, you aren't going to accomplish much.

2. The afterburn effect is greatly overrated, accounting for maybe an additional 10% calorie burn after the workout. Considering you could burn a few hundred calories during the HIIT session, I wouldn't get too excited about burning 20-30 more calories afterward.

3. If performed with sufficient intensity, HIIT causes nervous system fatigue, just like intense weightlifting. Therefore, you must recover from it just like weightlifting. If you perform HIIT one day, then lift weights the next day, back-and-forth, you will find yourself in an over-trained state pretty quickly.

4. If you perform a high-volume weight training session with short rest breaks, it basically is performing HIIT. You will even notice an EPOC effect that can last long after a hard gym session. For my money, I'd rather just lift weights then.

Some examples of HIIT exercises are:

- Calisthenics

- Sandbag training

- Giant sets

- Barbell Complexes

- Sprints

- Variable resistance stationary bike

For HIIT to be effective, the best tips I have are:

1. Go hard! I mean, leave it all on the field. If you're not panting into a pool of your own sweat, if you can feel your arms and legs, if you're not suffocating from lack of oxygen, then it's not HIIT.

2. Take less than 15 seconds between sets, which is really just the time it takes to switch exercises. There are no true rest breaks in HIIT.

LISS – Low Intensity, Steady State

This is the old school cardio you're used to, like jogging on a treadmill or riding a bike for miles-and-miles. The idea is to raise your heart rate and then keep it there. The real benefit of LISS is it burns fat as a primary fuel source because it's low effort. However, it burns it at a relatively slow pace because it doesn't take that much energy (i.e., calories) to perform. The more intense you perform the activity, the higher the calorie burn rate. But if you go too hard, you run into fatigue issues when you cross into HIIT territory. LISS must be performed for at least 20-minutes to matter, and in my opinion, at least 40-minutes to be worth doing at all.

Some examples of LISS exercises are:

- Jogging
- Swimming
- Elliptical
- Rowing
- Biking

Some bodybuilders use LISS when leading up to competition, mainly as a way to speed up fat burning. Keep in mind though that these are highly trained lifters who are likely on PEDs. It makes a big difference. If you're going to incorporate LISS into your program, you need to keep an eye on your calorie burn, or you could end up overdoing it and actually eating into your muscle mass.

Fasted vs. Fed Cardio

This is an old debate that I feel has been settled by real science, if not by "bro science." The idea that training first thing in the morning on an empty stomach burns more fat than cardio after you've eaten goes back to the 1970s, but really wasn't studied closely for a few decades after, allowing the idea to take deep root in gym lore. The thinking is that since your stomach is empty in the morning, your insulin and blood sugar levels will be low; therefore, your body is able to burn fat easily. Great idea. It turns out, in the long run, it doesn't matter if you do cardio before or after you eat. What matters is a long-term caloric deficit.

Fasted cardio always makes me feel weak and exhausted, throwing off my morning if not the whole day. Skip this bro-science myth and do cardio (if you must) to build cardiovascular health, not to burn fat.

Essential Takeaways

- Cardio for heart health and endurance makes sense. Cardio for fat loss, not so much.
- Cardio burns calories and requires recovery, both of which can hamper your gains.
- Perform less cardio during bulk cycles and more during cut cycles.

Chapter 8

REST, DELOAD, RECOVERY, AND INJURIES

Recovery Essentials

You don't grow in the gym. You grow while you rest. Rest is as crucial to growth as progressive overload and proper nutrition. We must rest daily, getting at least 7-hours of sleep, and take rest days weekly. You simply cannot exercise every day of the week and expect to grow muscle.

- **Rest** means sleeping and no movement above an easy walk.

Sufficient rest leads to growth. Insufficient rest leads to over-training syndrome. But there is a sweet spot in there because excessive rest leads to loss of adaptations and fat gain. Taking a few days off from the gym every week is correct. Taking weeks off at a time is not.

- **Deload** means exercising with reduced intensity and/or volume.

Rest means doing nothing. You're not resting if you're at the gym. Deloading means exercising with less intensity. This is something you might do if you're injured, excessively sore, or before a sporting event or competition. The idea is to move your body without truly taxing it. This is also a form of active recovery. The movement helps flush fresh blood into your muscles, speeding up recovery and allowing connective tissue to heal. It's a good idea to take a deload week once every couple of months.

Total Stress Management

When we exercise, we intentionally stress our bodies to encourage supercompensation. But our bodies are subject to more than just exercise-induced stress. Work, personal life, finances, disease, sickness, injuries, extreme temperatures, and many other factors contribute to our overall stress, and all of these combine to thwart our gains.

I am no guru of stress management and will freely admit that, as an entrepreneur in the boom or bust oil and gas industry, stress is a constant companion of mine. I have only learned one steadfast trick for overall stress management, and that is this:

Live by routine.

Routine is your friend. Routine allows you to get things done on autopilot. If you have to think about every little step you take each day, if every day is a new, unplanned experience, your stress levels will be through the roof. The more daily functions you can put on autopilot, the better.

The mantra I repeat to my trainees is simple, but powerful:

Set yourself up for success!

This means meal prepping on Sunday night, so you don't have to deal with it at 6:00am while you're trying to get yourself and kids out the door for school and work. It means leaving your headphones in your gym bag so you don't get to the gym and realize you forgot them at home. It means leaving your car keys in the exact same spot every day without fail, so you never have to hunt for them. Simply put, it means establishing the habit of doing things ahead of time so you can breeze through as much of your day as possible. You can't control everything that comes at you, so control the things you can, like simple daily activities, by consciously thinking of the best way to do things and then do it that way over-and-over again until it becomes a habit.

Over-training Syndrome

Over-training syndrome (OTS) is a condition you find yourself in when you have out-worked your body's ability to recover. When you train hard, rest little, under-nourish yourself, and then repeat, all the cumulative stress and damage to your body becomes too much for your body to handle. Systems start to underperform or even crash. OTS causes real stress to multiple bodily systems, including your neurologic, endocrinologic, and immunologic systems.

Some classic symptoms of OTS are:

- Amped-up, sleepless nights.

- Lack of energy and a general feeling of fatigue.

- Persistent strength plateaus.

- Lack of motivation in the gym.

- Persistent sinus or chest congestion and other infections that don't heal.

The best solution for OTS is prevention. If you suspect you may already be over-trained, the only solution is to take a week off from the gym (and all other strenuous activity), make sure your diet is on point, and get some real rest.

Cardio competes for resources (nutrients, calories, and rest) with the muscle repair operations your body must conduct after lifting weights. That same rule applies to every physical activity. If you play recreational sports, such as basketball, tennis, rock climbing, bicycling, etc., it's important that you realize those physical activities also tax your body. That means extracurricular activities count towards your maximum recoverable volume (MRV). If you plan to have a strenuous weekend, maybe take a deload week before and/or after. Give your body a chance to recuperate fully.

Here's the takeaway:

It's crucial to watch the bottom line, add up all your activities, and make sure you're not exceeding your ability to recover. The more active you are, the more quality rest and calories you will need.

Injuries

What's the age-old coach's prescription for injury? "Walk it off!" There is something to be said for active recovery, sure. But at the same time, you're not 14 anymore. At 40+ years old, I'm going to tell you to allow injuries to heal fully. If you don't, they will simply get worse-and-worse.

I have learned this through experience, and many older lifters will tell you the same. If your shoulder starts hurting during bench press, doing more bench press is most likely just going to make it worse. Aches and pains can stick around for months or years (or a lifetime) if you don't properly rest and rehab them.

A full discussion of every possible injury you might face is beyond the scope of this book. It is a topic best addressed by a physical therapist or doctor, anyway. For our purposes, pain means injury, and injuries must be rested.

If you think you strained a muscle or sprained a joint, follow the RICE protocol as soon as you get home to begin reducing inflammation as soon as possible.

Rice stands for:

- **Rest**: We've talked about this.

- **Ice**: Put an icepack inside a thin towel or t-shirt and apply it to the hurt area.

- **Compression**: Wrap the injured area in a compression bandage to prevent swelling.

- **Elevation**: Elevating an injury above your heart reduces throbbing and swelling.

After RICE, Ibuprofen and sleep are your best friends. Once the pain subsides, gentle stretching and massage can help speed recovery.

Here's the takeaway:

Unless instructed otherwise by a professional, do not attempt to work through an injury. Instead, allow it to heal by resting and performing exercises that don't use that muscle or joint for however many weeks it takes for the pain to stop.

Essential Takeaways

- Sleep at least 7 hours per night.

- Take rest days every week.

- Use deload days as needed.

- Manage total stress by implementing smart routines in your day.

- Use RICE, ibuprofen, massage, and physical therapy for injuries.

Chapter 9

EQUIPMENT

Equipment Essentials

Unless you're building a home gym, weightlifting does not require a lot of equipment. Most of what you need (weights) is covered by your gym membership. That said, a few items deserve special discussion:

- **Shoes**: Shoes with soft or air soles will compress under heavy weight, making lifts like the squat more difficult. On leg day or when performing deadlifts, wear shoes with a solid sole, such as Chuck Taylors, Vans, No Bull Trainers, or weightlifting shoes.

- **Weightlifting Belt:** A wide, leather weightlifting belt should be used during heavy, upright lifts such as squat and deadlift. Proper use of the weight belt requires learning the Valsalva maneuver, which you can look up online.

- **Lifting Straps:** Straps should be used during heavy, upright barbell lifts, such as the deadlift, when the load becomes too heavy for your grip. People will argue that straps are a crutch and that a "real lifter" will allow the barbell to strengthen their grip. There is some value to this, especially at relatively low weights. However, if my back can handle deadlifting 315-lbs, but my grip can't, it would be foolish to allow the weak link in the chain (my forearm muscles) to prevent me from getting a good back workout. Plus, if you've never had medial epicondylitis, also known as "golfer's elbow," you don't want it. Golfer's elbow can be caused when a heavy weight slips from your grip down into your fingers instead of deep in your palm. This puts incredible strain on a thin, weak muscle that attaches to the inside of your elbow and runs out to your fingers. This muscle is not meant to support hundreds of pounds, so it will strain easily. Once it's strained, gripping anything will become painful, and you'll have to adjust your workout or take time off. Use the straps and avoid injuries.

- **Headphones**: There is no doubt in my mind that listening to the music that moves you will increase your performance and make your gym sessions more enjoyable, as most gyms play horrible music.

- **Gym bag**: I carry my gym bag around with me and use it to mark my territory. I don't hog equipment, but I do pace between sets. Putting my bag under the bench or next to the machine I'm using makes it clear to others that the station is taken, thus avoiding the whole "Are you using that?" conversation. Make sure the bag is large enough to fit not just your basic gear but also your weight belt, hoodie, water bottle, and shaker.

- **Multiple hand towels**: A hand towel is always useful. Sweat has bacteria in it, so if you leave a dirty towel in your gym bag, it will be funky within hours. Therefore, unless you plan to wash your one towel several times a week, keep a few towels around so you'll always have a clean one until you can wash them all.

- **Water bottles**: I just refill the same single-use water bottle until it gets funky.

- **Multiple shakers**: The iconic BlenderBottle with the wire ball is still the best way to mix supplement shakes. The thing is, whey and casein are milk proteins and milk spoils. If you don't wash your shakers immediately after use, they will smell awful. I keep no less than 10 shakers around. Every day after the gym, I rinse the shaker I used well and put it in the dishwasher to get sterilized once I run it. The next day, I pull a totally clean one from the cabinet. Trying to keep one shaker properly washed all the time is not practical, at least not for me.

- **Hand sanitizer**: Staph infections can spread at gyms.

- **Resistance bands**: These are optional but cheap and useful.

- **Running shoes**: Hard-soled weightlifting shoes are not suitable for running, so if you plan to do cardio, you'll need appropriate running shoes. I have suffered from shin splints for a long time, making jogging a real pain. Some years ago, I had a gait analysis done and bought the running shoes recommended for my feet. Immediately, my distance doubled. Good running shoes are worth it, and the latest big brand shoes off the shelf might not be right for you.

- **Wrist wraps**: Some guys like wrist wraps for bench press and other lifts. I don't use them, but they may be something that helps you. If you have wrist pain, try them out.

- **Knee wraps**: The purpose of knee wraps is not really to brace your knee. They're too flimsy for that. Their main purpose is to keep your knees warm to prevent tendon and ligament damage. Use them if it makes sense for you.

- **Bathroom scale**: A basic bathroom scale is necessary.

- **Food scale.**

- **Measuring cup.**

Chapter 10

PROGRESS TRACKING

Tracking Essentials

How do you know if you're making progress if you're not tracking anything? But how often and what should you be tracking? Tracking is important, but it's also important not to obsess over it.

I advise my trainees to weigh and measure themselves once per week on an empty stomach, on the same day, and at the same time every week. In my house, Tuesday morning is weigh-in day. I have a bathroom scale, tape measure, and a chart and pen thumb tacked to the wall. Hit the head, strip down, take your weight, measure your limbs and torso. Everything gets recorded on the chart. It takes about 3-minutes. The same chart I have tacked to my bathroom wall is included at the end of this book for your use.

There is no single measurement device that gives you a complete picture of your physique (though a DEXA scan plus a 3D body scan comes really close). Use a combination of tools to get a complete picture, but most of all, be patient. Change comes, but in months and years, not days or weeks.

- **Fitness journals** are used by many lifters to keep track of their workouts, the weight they lifted, and the number of sets and reps performed. There are many ways to track workouts, from spiral notebooks to smartphone apps. Personally, I only keep track of my 5RMs for the big, compound joint lifts (deadlift, bench press, squat, overhead press) using the Notes app on my iPhone. Everything else, I either have it logged in my head, or I just lift by feel. You should think about a fitness journaling method that works for you.

- **MyFitnessPal** is a fantastic tool for tracking. I use it to track my body weight, and I upload mirror selfies of myself every so often.

- **DEXA scans** are also great but cost a few dollars, so they are better to perform every 6 months or so.

- **Photos** are the best way to track progress, I think. Set a repeating alert in your calendar and take a new progress photo every month.

- **A bathroom scale** is a useful tool but can also be frustrating. Am I losing fat and gaining muscle? Am I retaining water? Is the scale broken? Use the scale as a long-term tracking tool, not something you obsess about every pound over.

- **A tape measure**, the kind that tailors or seamstresses use, is useful. Measure the circumference of one upper arm, one thigh, your waist, chest, and neck. Measure around the same place every time. On your upper arms and thighs, make sure to go around the thickest part. On your waist, measure around your belly button.

- **An old pair of jeans** that used to fit you perfectly or a current pair of "fat jeans" that will fit you more loosely as you drop pounds can provide a great 3-dimensional measure of weight loss. But as your thighs get bigger and your waist smaller, you may find those old pants don't fit you anymore.

Chapter 11

SUMMARY

A quick recap of how to organize your program:

- Begin by building solid training habits and a routine you can adhere to for months or years.

- If your initial goal is to lose body fat (most of you), begin with a cut cycle.

- Reduce calories, intensity, and volume during a cut.

- Perform PPL or other higher volume, moderate weight programs during a cut.

- You can increase cardio during a cut, but be careful not to over exhaust yourself.

- Once your weight loss plateaus, gradually switch to a bulk cycle.

- During a bulk, increase calories, intensity, and volume.

- To gain strength during a bulk, work in the 3-5RM range. For hypertrophy, work in the 10RM range.

- Bulk until you hit a strength plateau or accumulate excessive body fat (over 20%), then switch back to a cut cycle.

- Cycle between strength and hypertrophy programs, back and forth, every 6-12 weeks.

- Take a deload or rest week between cycles.

- Avoid injuries at all costs.

- Be patient and consistent.

- Above all else, do not quit!

There is a reason trainers and fitness pros call the process of getting in-shape a journey. As you have learned, gaining strength and muscle is not a simple, straightforward process. Between your current body and the body you envision, there will be ups-and-downs. There will be days when you crush personal records and feel like a god and days when your body doesn't cooperate. There will be injuries that seem unfair, soreness, life changes, and innumerable distractions. When you find yourself discouraged, picture your goal, and remember to have faith in your routine. Build healthy habits, and encourage yourself always to push and evolve into the best person you can be.

I hope the knowledge you've gained this book sparks a new motivation in you, and that you will work every day to build strong new habits and a strong new body.

Remember:

There is no improvement inside the comfort zone!

If you enjoyed this book, please leave me a review on Amazon. As a new writer, it's very difficult to get eyes on my books. Reviews from readers help bring more attention, so please consider leaving me a review.

Thank you and be sure to keep in touch!

www.rexhollowaywriter.com

Reddit: u/RexHollowayWriter

X: @writer_rex4235

YouTube: @RexHolloway

Sample Hypertrophy Program

	MONDAY	TUESDAY	WEDNESDAY	THURSDAY	FRIDAY	SATURDAY	SUNDAY
PUSH-PULL-LEGS HYPERTROPHY SPLIT	PUSH	REST	LEGS	REST	PULL	REST	REST
	Warmup 5-minutes on treadmill 10-minutes stretching Chest 3 x 10 - Flat dumbbell bench 3 x 10 - Incline Dumbbell bench 3 x 10 - Dips 3 x 10 - Cable crossover Shoulders 3 x 10 - Standing dumbbell shoulder press (single arm) 3 x 10 - Standing dumbbell lateral raise (single arm) 3 x 10 - Face pulls Triceps 3 x 10 - Overhead dumbbell triceps extension 3 x 10 - Cable triceps pushdown Abs 3 x to failure - Lower ab leg raises 3 x to failure - Crunches 3 x to failure - Woodchoppers with band Cool Down 5-minutes walking on the treadmill		Warmup 5-minutes on treadmill 10-minutes stretching Legs 3 x 10 - Barbell squats 3 x 10 - Stiff-legged dead lift 3 x 10 - Smith Machine Split squats 3 x 10 - Dumbbell lunges 3 x 10 - Standing calf-raises 3 x 10 - Seated calf-raises Cool Down 5-minutes walking on the treadmill		Warmup 5-minutes on treadmill 10-minutes stretching Back 3 x 10 - Pull-ups or Lat pull 3 x 10 - Straight-arm Pulldown 3 x 10 - Seated row 3 x 10 - Face pulls Biceps 3 x 10 - Alternating dumbbell curls Abs 3 x to failure - Lower ab leg raises 3 x to failure - Crunches 3 x to failure - Woodchoppers with band Cool Down 5-minutes walking on the treadmill		

Sample Strength Program

	MONDAY	TUESDAY	WEDNESDAY	THURSDAY	FRIDAY	SATURDAY	SUNDAY
5x5 TRAINING SPLIT	PUSH	REST	LEGS	REST	PULL	REST	REST
	<u>Warmup</u> 5-minutes on treadmill 10-minutes stretching 5 x 5 – Barbell squat 5 x 5 – Barbell bench press 5 x 5 – Bent-over barbell row 3 x 10 – Barbell curls <u>Abs</u> 3 x to failure - Lower ab leg raises 3 x to failure - Crunches 3 x to failure - Woodchoppers with band <u>Cool Down</u> 5-minutes walking on the treadmill		<u>Warmup</u> 5-minutes on treadmill 10-minutes stretching 5 x 5 – Barbell overhead press 5 x 5 – Barbell deadlift 5 x 5 – Lat pull 3 x 10 – Lateral shoulder raises <u>Abs</u> 3 x to failure - Lower ab leg raises 3 x to failure - Crunches 3 x to failure - Woodchoppers with band <u>Cool Down</u> 5-minutes walking on the treadmill		<u>Warmup</u> 5-minutes on treadmill 10-minutes stretching 5 x 5 – Barbell squat 5 x 5 – Barbell bench press 5 x 5 – Bent-over barbell row 3 x 10 – Dips <u>Abs</u> 3 x to failure - Lower ab leg raises 3 x to failure - Crunches 3 x to failure - Woodchoppers with band <u>Cool Down</u> 5-minutes walking on the treadmill		

Sample Nutrition Plan

ITEM	QTY	CALORIES	PROTEIN	CARBS	FATS
BREAKFAST					
Eggs, lg	2	143	12.6	0.7	9.5
Oatmeal	0.5 cup	150	5	27	3
Walnuts	15	200	5	4	20
Blueberries	10	8	0	2	0
TOTALS		**503**	**22.6**	**33.7**	**32.5**
LUNCH					
Sirloin, lean	8 oz	514	60	0	29
Green beans, steamed	1 cup	53	2.7	10.7	0
TOTALS		**567**	**62.7**	**10.7**	**29**
AFTERNOON SNACK					
Whey protein	1 scoop	120	24	3	1
Water	12 oz	0	0	0	0
TOTALS		**120**	**24**	**3**	**1**
PRE-WORKOUT SHAKE					
Whey protein	0.5 scoop	60	12	1.5	0.5
Pre-Workout	0.5 scoop	10	0	2	0
Water	12 oz	0	0	0	0
TOTALS		**70**	**12**	**3.5**	**0.5**
POST-WORKOUT SHAKE					
Whey protein	1 scoop	120	24	3	1
Creatine	1 serv	0	0	0	0
Dextrose	1 scoop	190	0	47	0
Water	12 oz	0	0	0	0
TOTALS		**310**	**24**	**50**	**1**
DINNER					
Grilled salmon	6 oz	150	31.5	3	1.5
Green beans, steamed	1 cup	53	2.7	10.7	0
White rice	1 cup	205	4	45	0
TOTALS		**408**	**38.2**	**58.7**	**1.5**
PRE-BEDTIME SHAKE					
Casein protein	1 scoop	120	24	3	1
Fat-free milk	12 oz	135	13.5	19.5	0
TOTALS		**255**	**37.5**	**22.5**	**1**
		CALORIES	**PROTEIN**	**CARBS**	**FATS**
TOTALS		2,233	221g	182g	67g

Sample Tracking Chart

WEEK	DATE	CYCLE	WEIGHT	ARMS	CHEST	THIGHS	WAIST	NECK	NOTES
1									
2									
3									
4									
5									
6									
7									
8									
9									
10